History
of Energy
Transference

History of Energy Transference

Exploring the Foundations of Modern Healing

Willy Schrödter

SAMUEL WEISER, INC.

York Beach, Maine

First published in 1999 by
Samuel Weiser, Inc.
P. O. Box 612
York Beach, ME 03910-0612
www.weiserbooks.com

Library of Congress Cataloging-in-Publication Data

Schrödter, Willy, 1897–1971.
   [Präsenzwirkung. English]
   History of energy transference : exploring the foundations of modern healing / Willy Schrödter.
      p.   cm.
   Includes bibliographical references and index.
   ISBN 1–57863–101–7 (pbk. : alk. paper)
   1. Parapsychology.   2. Spiritual healing.   I. Title.
BF1033.S32513   1999
615.8′52—dc21   98-53594
                                                          CIP
MV

Translated by Transcript, Ltd.

Typeset in Palatino

Printed in the United States of America

07 06 05 04 03 02 01 00 99
10 9 8 7 6 5 4 3 2 1

Contents

For human beings no remedy is better than
another human being.

—Petrus Blesenius
(1135–1200 [?])

Of all the bodies in nature it is the human
being that acts most efficiently on humans.

—Dr. F. A. Mesmer
(1733–1815)

Even when passive, humans seem to emanate
a perceptible ambient force.

—Dr. Gérard A. Van Rijnberk
(1875–1953) *"Les Métasciences
biologiques* "Adyar" [Paris]
1952, p. 104

If you can cheer up an unhappy soul by the
power of your words of comfort, by a friendly
look, or even perhaps by your mere presence,
that is a magical act.

—Dr. Franz Hartmann
(1838–1912) "Magic and
Occult Science," *Occult
World*, Rochester, NY,
November, 1887

for he has renounced everything we call personality. He has concentrated on God for forty years . . . and by doing so has unceasingly served humanity, especially the poor. . . . Sant Mota had the
gift of clairvoyance but did not exploit it, and basically wished to
work through nothing apart from his *power-packed radiation*" (Prof.
Gebhard FREI, "Christian Mantra-Yoga: The Prayer of the Heart,"
Meditation in Religion and Psychotherapy, Stuttgart, 1958).

This is one case where a phenomenon originating in the
moral plane is transferred to the physical plane. "The human
being as a whole transcends the reach of medicine" (Dr. Erich
STIEFVATER, *The Mind's Eye*, Ulm/Donau, 1957).

At his most effective, a healer of this kind is a healer "by the
grace of God," he or she is not the almighty factor but only the willing tool of the Higher Power (DRESSER). In other words, the healer is
one who is continually giving out and continually being refilled as
a vessel that opens itself to the Transcendent (Ps. 81:11; Mt. 11: 25).

Such a "vessel" becomes legitimate when diseases are repeatedly cured within a short space of time without medicaments or
other therapeutic means. The healer acts as a transformer of
macrocosmic and metacosmic forces (just as official medicine is
able to do with its remedies) and this "relayer of the Transcendent" may quite successfully alleviate illness even if the patient
eventually succumbs to it.

I find an allusion to this distant goal in a pronouncement by
Ralph Waldo TRINE:

"The time will come when the work of the physician will not
be to treat and attempt to heal the body, but to heal the mind,
which in turn will heal the body." *In Tune with the Infinite* (London: G. Bell & Sons Ltd. (reprint) 1918), p. 77.

To some extent, the silent transmission of our inner radiant
power, which is able to stimulate the *vis medicatrix naturae* [the
healing power of nature] may rightly be practiced in private by
those who are morally developed, in the "inmost heart" (Japanese: *hara*) of their calm healing personality; but in any case it is an
imponderable something that ought to accompany every remedy. And the more one is aware of it the more readily will it flow.
However, in that higher grade where it is the sole agent (i.e., is
employed exclusively) such "spiritual" healing is subject to the
condition that, in general, it cannot be reproduced like a mechanical technique or science.

Introduction

From time to time we need, as it were, to be "rebound" by consorting with those who are good and strong; otherwise we shall lose a few pages.
—F. W. NIETZSCHE *(1844–1900)*

There have been exceptional individuals in every time and place who have the natural ability to exercise a healthy (beneficial to body and spirit) or unhealthy (prejudicial to body and spirit) influence on their surroundings, *through their mere, silent, outwardly inactive presence.*

In keeping with the convention of RHINE, who labeled parapsychological phenomena with the word *psi* and the names of other Greek letters (*gamma, kappa*), we could call our present subject the *Psi-pi*-phenomenon (where *pi* stands for *parousia*, the Greek for "presence").

The purpose of our study is to investigate the causes, the effects, and where possible the therapeutic implications of this phenomenon.

It will become clear from our analysis that this influencing of third parties arises out of both physical and psychic elements or conditions. Usually both occur together, and in such a way that the psychic (emotional) agent—as obviously superordinate—infiltrates, saturates, deneutralizes, and modifies the physical (corporeal) emanations! Therefore the power of the influence depends primarily on the intensity of the emotions, which in the therapeutic sector means a constantly renewed, burning desire to help (cf. Jn. 9: 33, 35, 38). Thus a decisive factor is the moral suffering of the influencer, which will probably be more exalted the more humble the individual ego is. The Indian swami, Ram Das, tells of a 60-year-old Indian, Sant Mota, who lived in Gujerat. His devotees called him simply "my brother." Few knew him. He helped many by what he wrote. Ram Das says of him, "In personal intercourse he operates with nothing at all. A piercing nothing issues from him,

INFLUENCE BY PHYSICAL PRESENCE

> *You are a very disturbing magnet. . . . I believe to a certain extent in magnetism . . . but I have never accepted the idea that persons can silently and almost without conscious effort, influence others for malign or beneficial purposes. In your presence, however, the thing is forced upon me as though it were a truth . . .*
>
> *—Marie CORELLI*[1]

In the cultural history of all times and places there are records of people who merely by their *quiet and outwardly inactive presence* have been able to exercise a healthy or unhealthy influence on their surroundings. The word "inactive" immediately alerts us to the fact that what we have here is not the taking of a lead when an opportunity arises, but "contagion" with the essential radiation of a personality possessing a certain psychic structure.

Agrippa von NETTESHEIM (1486–1535) put it this way in 1510: "Even as asafoetida and musk drench everything in their smell, so something evil is imparted to their neighbors by the evil and something good by the good, and often it clings to them for a long time."[2]

EXTREMELY PSYCHOACTIVE PEOPLE

I have deliberately refrained from using the words "strong personalities," because some people who have a negative effect on their environment are the exact opposite of this, and what they

---

[1]CORELLI, Marie, *The Life Everlasting* (New York: Grosset & Dunlap, 1911), p. 294.
[2]v. NETTESHEIM, Agrippa, *Occult Philosophy*, Bk. I (Antwerp, 1510), chapter 65.

do is confined to paralyzing others and leeching them of their vitality; for which reason Dr. Eugène Osty, (1874–1938) called them "personnes stérilisantes." Now even if our examples were only of people like this, it would be reasonable to infer the existence of their opposites, whom the Budapest medical hypnotist Dr. Franz Völgyesi in 1941 labeled "extremely psychoactive" individuals.[3]

THE EVIL EYE—"OCULAR RAYS"

Some cases of the so-called *evil eye* (Italian *jettatura, mal occhio*),[4] the existence of which is widely accepted by educated people, especially in Italy, might easily be explained as the negative effect of the whole personality; nevertheless modern researchers do assign a decisive role to the malign glance[5] of the *jettatore* [person possessing an evil eye],[6] and an electroscopic apparatus made in England is said to have been deflected by rays emitted from the eye.[7]

Dr. Walter Voeller (1893–1954) claims to have demonstrated with his *Organoelectrometer* that "continual neural-electrical discharges are emitted from the eyes."[8] German mesmerists have taken great pains to demonstrate by simple means the *émission pésante* or "ponderable emission" from the human eye.[9]

[3]Völgyesi, Dr. Franz, *Min den a lélek* (Budapest, 1941); *Die Seele ist alles* [The Mind is All] (Zürich, 1948), p. 26

[4]Seligmann, Dr. Siegfried, *Der Böse Blick und Verwandtes* (The Evil Eye and Related Matters] (Berlin, 1910); *Die Zauberkraft des Auges und das Berufen* [The Wizardry of the Eye and the Vocation] (Hamburg, 1922).

[5]Matthew's Gospel 6: 22–23.

[6]Müller, Alexander, *Sepdelenopathie* (Bad Kreuznach, 1921), p. 15; Clarence, E.W., "Sympathie, Mumia, Amulette, okk. Kräfte der Edelsteine und Metalle" [Sympathy, Mummy, Amulets, Occult Powers of Gems and Metals] *Okkulte Medizin*, Bd. XII, 1, S. 7; Tanagras, Angelos, M.D., *Le Destin et la Chance* [Destiny and Chance] Athens, Société des Recherches psych.

[7]Memminger, Anton, "Hakenkreuz und Davidstern" [Swastika and Magen David], *Volkstüml. Einführg. i.d. Geh. Wissenschaften* [A Popular Introduction to the Occult Sciences] (Würzburg, 1922), pp. 221–222.

[8]Voeller, Dr. Walter, "Neue Anschauungen über Hypnose, Suggestion und Telepathie" [A New Approach to Hypnosis, Suggestion and Telepathy], *Z. Heilmagnetismus* (1926), 8 [November] : 58 f.

[9]Schabenberger, Johann, *Das Wesen des Heilmagnetismus* [The Nature of Healing Magnetism] (Munich, 1906), p. 12 f; Breitung, Max, *Heilmagnetismus in der Familie* [Healing Magnetism in the Family] (Leipzig, 1924), p. 42, 6.

At all events, Charles LAFONTAINE, one of the most notable mesmerists of a century ago, reported several cases of the killing of small animals within a quarter of an hour by the gaze, while each time the experimenter suffered from unpleasant recoil reactions (weakness, headache, smarting eyes).[10]

The "most unlikely jettatore known" in recent times was Cardinal Pignatelli DI BELMONTE (1851–1948), if the usually well-informed Roger PEYREFITTE is to be believed.[11]

THE THEME IN LITERATURE

Literature has often seized on our subject. Here we have space only for a passing reference to the declaration of GOETHE's Margarethe in regard to Dr. Heinrich FAUST's companion Mephistopheles:

"His presence agitates my blood."[12]
"And his presence stifles me inside."[13]

---

[10]LAFONTAINE, Charles, *L'Art de magnétiser ou le Magnétisme animal* [The Art of Mesmerism or Animal Magnetism] (Paris, 1860), pp. 331–336.

[11]PEYREFITTE, Roger, *Die Schlüssel von St. Peter* [St. Peter's Keys] (Karlsruhe, 1956), p. 221 f.

[12]v. GOETHE, J.W., *Faust* (Reclams Universal Bibliothek), First Part (Leipzig, n.d.), scene 16, line 3477.

[13]*Faust*, l. c., line 3493.

SYMPATHY, ANTIPATHY, INDIFFERENCE

There is certainly something in the law of attraction between human beings which we do not understand.
—*Marie* CORELLI[14]

This sentence from an imaginative writer, who often "know more than the philosophic head" (that is to say, who on the basis of what reason derides as "unreliable intuition" arrives sooner and more often than reason does at valuable perceptions—which, naturally, will have to be presented in a rational dress to the rank and file who have little or no intuition) this word, I say, brings us at a stroke to the common experience of being affected by another person. For in most of us in whom the parasitic cerebrum[15] has still not quite overrun the emotions, there arises, on meeting a stranger, a feeling that immediately allows us to differentiate between compatible, attractive, *sympathetic* individuals and incompatible, unattractive, *antipathetic* individuals. After spending more time with them we can also speak of those who are "a tonic" to us and those who are "wet blankets." In addition there are those in the majority who are neutral or *indifferent*.

Everyday life repeatedly teaches us that later experience will usually confirm the initial emotional judgment that is often flatly opposed to the intellectual judgment.

Here is an example from the medical sector: the celebrated internist, CHVOSTEK made the following observation: "When I first examine a patient I suddenly become aware of the nature of the disease as if by inspiration. Then, on completing the usual tests, I

[14]CORELLI: *The Life Everlasting*, p. 291.
[15]KLAGES, Ludwig, *Der Geist als Widersacher de Seele* [The Mind as an Adversary of the Soul] (1929–1932); SEIDEL, Alfred, *Bewußtsein als Verhängnis* [Consciousness as Fate] (Bonn, 1927); THIESS, Frank, *Despotie des Intellekts* [The Despotism of the Intellect] (Kassel, 1949).

reach a completely different conclusion. In the process of time, often after several weeks, the accuracy of my *instantaneous initial diagnosis* is confirmed."[16]

The guardian of Kaspar HAUSER (1812 [?]–1833), Baron Gottlieb VON TUCHER (a member of the Kreisrat), wrote to the professor of Evangelical Theology, Dr. August THOLUCK (1799–1877) in Halle a.d.S., as published by the latter in his *Literarischen Anzeiger für christliche Theologie und Wissenschaft* (1840, 318–320): "The effect that people had on him (Hauser) varied greatly; being pleasant or unpleasant, and in debauches was foul and disgusting even though he knew nothing of their way of life. Each individual has—said he—a personal scent, *though it is not the kind that is smelled by the nose but quite different*. He could not find words to describe it."[17]

One is reminded of a comment that the Viennese "psychological dietician" Baron Ernst VON FEUCHTERSLEBEN (1806–1849) apparently quoted from Karl Leberecht IMMERMANN (1796–1840): "It is a pity that we do not know if the noted Berlin physician Dr. HEIM, who was so renowned a diagnostician and could accurately distinguish between various cutaneous eruptions by their smell, could also sniff out moral proclivities by the same organ."

PERSONAL SCENT—THE ODOR OF SANCTITY

There may in fact be *occasional subliminal* odorific stimuli involved in the emotional interaction between two individuals. As an illustration of being "in evil odor" here is a quotation from the physician August STRINDBERG (1849–1912). In an attempt to reify the indefinable, he says: "If someone smells of rats, he is a skinflint . . . hatred smells like a corpse." Proverbially there is an (agreeable) "odor of sanctity," which can be taken literally. Among many other things, holiness is based on sexual abstinence. JOYCE puts the following apposite monologue in the mouth of his character *Bloom*:

---

[16]THETTER, Rudolf, *Magnetismus—das Urheilmittel* [Magnetism—The Original Curative Agent] (Vienna, 1951), p. 119.

[17]M.W., *Kaspar Hauser—die Kräfte des unverdorbenen natürlichen Menschen* ["The Faculties of Unsophisticated People"], Sphinx (1888), 29 May: 346.

> *Perhaps they [the female sex] get a smell off us . . . must be*
> *connected with that because priests that are supposed to be are*
> *different. Women buzz round it like flies round treacle. . . .*
> *That diffuses itself all through the body, permeates. Source of*
> *life and it's extremely curious the smell. Celery sauce."[18]*

He is seconded by a well-known pendulist researching the *odic* side of the question: "The male seed contains very powerful odic forces, and the pendulum describes the most lively circles over it. . . . Its radiations pervade the whole body, and after a seminal emission this influence in the body falls to a minimum. A sensitive man will perceive the diminution in radiation. A young husband who is sowing unsparingly in the garden of love can always be recognized by his feeble radiations. . . . A man with a good store of radiant power is unusually attractive to a sensitive woman and she is easily won."[19]

And "easily won" describes the three ladies in GOETHE'S *Faust* when they caught a whiff of the man Paris (*Faust*, Part Two, Act I, lines 6473–6479, Reclam).

According to the esoteric Tantric document *Bhairavi Diksha*, retained sexual energy is sublimated into a subtle essence, *ojas*, which is stored in the brain.[20] And according to another textbook of Yoga (Svâtmaramâ, *Hathayogapradipika*, III, p. 89) it produces "a pleasant odor."

---

[18]JOYCE, James, *Ulysses* II (Basel, 1927), p. 343.

[19]GLAHN, A. Frank, *Glahns Pendelbücherei* [Glahn's Dowser's Library] V (Memmingen, 1931), p. 118.

[20]BIRVEN, Dr. Cl. Henri, *Lebenskunst in Yoga und Magie* [The Art of Living in Yoga and Magic] (Zürich, 1953), p. 66.

THE SOURCE OF
OUR IMPRESSIONS?

Similarly the appearance of individuals excites in us sympathy, love, or hate. But do not these various feelings come from the vibrations that emanate from these folk?
—G. LAKHOVSKY[21]

On what *ex*pression (imprinted from inside to outside) does our *im*pression of the person who confronts us depend? Proverbially, "first impressions are best"; which means that it is preferable to rely on those that have not been filtered through the brain.

DEDUCTIVE IMPRESSIONS

The most lasting impressions are based on what we infer from the forms of expression—the style of behavior of those we meet. Deduction is a purely intellectual function, and as such lies outside the scope of our present study.

PARTLY INSTINCTIVE IMPRESSIONS

Another way in which we form impressions of those we meet relies on externals, such as deportment, gesture, mimicry, manner of speaking (accent), handshake,[22] and physiognomy; of which

[21]LAKHOVSKY, Georges, *Das Geheimnis des Lebens* [The Secret of Life] (Munich, 1931), p. 243.
[22]ZEISS, Max, "Der Händedruck" [The Handshake], *Zbl. Okk.* 12926, 12 [June], 552 f.

the "cherubic wanderer" ANGELUS SILESIUS (Joh. Scheffler [1624–1677] sings:

> It is a righteous law on earth,
> That faces show their owners' worth.

And in the face it is the eyes that are "the light of the body" (Matt. 6:22) and they arrest us by their gaze.

In a variety of ways, this outer revelation of the inner prompts us by reflex action—so to speak—to make a *relationship judgment* (i.e., an assessment of the degree to which the other person is in tune with us), a judgment which quite often becomes verbal. My use of the words "reflex action" is meant to indicate that we are dealing here much more with the obtrusion on us of a person's outer form than with a regular, actual, physiognomical observation and examination carried out by our primary consciousness. It is something that lies between instinct and intellect, but somewhat nearer to instinct.

To this (and the next) section, a word may be added from Dr. Herbert MÜLLER-GUTTENBRUNN (d. 1945)—"the Lichtenberg of the 20th century"—in an old number of "Das Nebelhorn" [The Foghorn] (Vienna): "As little as I regard physiognomy as a science, so much do I believe in *intuitive* character reading *at first sight*."

WHOLLY INSTINCTIVE IMPRESSIONS

However, external appearances make the above-mentioned impression on us only if they are genuine, only if they are really expressing essential traits. If they are merely a pose, the partner's heart is known by its formless feelings and appearances are ignored! The transition from half-instinctive to fully instinctive face reading is made automatically: the presence of the other person is what matters.

After writing the above, I found the following corroboration of my explanation: Dr. Walter KRÖNER (then of Berlin-Charlottenburg) stated to an interviewer:

Each immediate psychological reaction to people and things: sympathy *and antipathy, liking and aversion, everything we understand by the notions presentiment, intuition, and* instinct, *does not spring naked from the pondering provoked by stimulation of the senses, or from association, but is at least partly the result of a direct, i.e.,* telepathic, *response. This intuitive reaction is especially striking in artists, women, and children. Hence, even in normal individuals, an* atavistic mediumistic ability *is continually at work in the unconscious.*[23]

But what is obtained by those who are naturally gifted is a representative cross-section of the essential nature of the partner crystallized from their thoughts, words, and deeds, and verified by later experience!

The Rosicrucian Trismegistus IV advised people to use this instinct:

Antipathies also form a part of magic (falsely) so-called. Man naturally has the same instinct as the animals; which warns them involuntarily against the creatures that are hostile or fatal to their existence. But he so often neglects it that it becomes dormant. Not so the true cultivator of the great science, etc.[24]

He has been seconded more recently (in 1923) by the self-initiated Gustav Meyrink (1868–1932):

In cases where the intellect alone is not sufficient for making a correct choice of the ways that should be taken, we must turn to our prescience and inner sensitivity while strengthening our instinct progressively, as if it were a compass needle we were learning to trust.[25]

---

[23]Zeiz, A.H., *Die Okkultisten: Propheten in deutscher Krise. Das Wunderbare od. die Verzauberten* [The Occultists: Prophets in a German crisis. The Supernatural or the Magical]. An anthology edited by Rudolf Olden (Berlin, 1932), p. 244.

[24]Bulwer, Edward, *Zanoni*; motto at head of chapter 8, Bk. I.

[25]Meyrink, Gustav, *An der Grenze des Jenseits* [On the Borders of the Other World] (Leipzig, 1923), p. 64.

REASON AND INSTINCT ANTAGONISTIC!

In this connection, Dr. Franz HARTMANN (1838–1912) admonishes us as follows:

> *What does a modern botanist know about the* signatures *of plants, by which the occultist recognizes the medicinal and occult properties of plants as soon as he sees them? The animals have remained natural, while man has become unnatural. The sheep does not need to be instructed by a zoologist to seek to escape if a tiger approaches: it knows by his signature and without argumentation that he is its enemy. Is it not more important for the sheep to know the ferocious character of the tiger than to be informed that the latter belongs to the genus* felis? *If by some miracle a sheep should become intellectual, it might learn so much about the external form, anatomy, physiology, and genealogy of the tiger, that it would lose sight of its internal character and be devoured by it.*[26]

This authority has a supporter in Prof. August BIER (1861–1949), privy councillor, who once said: "Man has become a farm animal with too much understanding and too little instinct."

On reading of HARTMANN's imaginary sheep which has become so intellectual that its inner eye is clouded, we are reminded of MEYRINK's instructive tale about a toad asking a millipede how it manages to keep leg pairs 1 and 2 in marching order with leg pairs 144 and 145, etc. The arthropod (which in fact never has more than 200 feet) tries to figure it out "and can no longer put one foot in front of another."[27]

---

[26]HARTMANN, Dr. Franz, *Ein Abenteuer unter Rosenkreuzern* (Leipzig, n.d., ca. 1912). English version, *An Adventure among the Rosicrucians* (Boston: The Occult Publishing Co., 1887). [Willy SCHRÖDTER omits HARTMANN's first sentence; but the reference to the old doctrine of signatures (according to which, for example, walnuts are good for our brains because they look like them) is not so clear without it. Therefore it has been inserted here. *Translator's note.*]

[27]MEYRINK, Gustav, *Der Flucht der Kröte; Des deutschen Spießers Wunderhorn* [The Toad's Curse: From The Plain German's Wonder Book] (Munich, 1948) p. 332; SEIDEL, 88.

Another parable introduces a man with a "doormat" of a beard who is asked by some impudent fellow whether he puts the beard over or under the blanket at night. The long-beard has a good long think and eventually replies. "With the best will in the world I cannot tell you. I myself do not know, for I have never noticed it." However, from then on, whenever the old man tried to go to sleep, he laid his beard on top of the blanket and this did not seem right; then he tucked it underneath and found this intolerable. What he used to do quite naturally had become a problem once he was aware of it! Just as the night-prowling troll overtaken by the first rays of the sun is petrified, so our vital automatism is disabled when brought into the light of consciousness!

WAVE TRANSMISSION

When there is no direct physical contact between two silent partners, it is obvious that the mediation of an instinctive impression can take place only by undulatory waves, so that the transference is like a radio transmission. Here is a prevailing unanimity of opinion on this subject from that of the "demonic knight" (ARAM) of Nettesheim through that of the saga writer Hermann Eris BUSSE (1891–1947). The former declared in 1510: "A foreign soul has no less power over the body of another than a foreign body has. Hence, we may assume, one individual acts on another *simply through temperament and character. . ."*

This is why the philosophers issue warnings against mixing with ill-natured and unfortunate people, as *their souls, filled with harmful rays,* infect their surroundings in a malign way. On the contrary, one should seek the company of good and fortunate people, since these *by their proximity* can be very profitable to us."[2] The latter asserted in 1939: "There are *rays* and *reverse rays* passing between individuals; so much is certain. Inexplicable antipathies and inexplicable attractions are caused by them."[28]

---

[2]See original footnote, p. 1.
[28]BUSSE, Hermann, *Erdgeist* [The Earth Spirit] (Leipzig, 1939), p. 322.

Biological Emanations or Thought-Waves?—"Od"

The question now arises: What can be the nature of these rays—
are they biological emanations or thought waves? In the middle
of the last century, Baron Karl von Reichenbach (1788–1869) identified, chiefly in human subjects, a fluid he called Od,[29] concerning which he left behind nine mostly bulky tomes. "Since he
made some 12,000 tests of the most varied sort, and under strin-
gent conditions, on about 150 persons of all classes, whoever
reads his writings will, if ready to feel the total impact of what
Reichenbach did, regard the existence of Od as established as sat-
isfactorily as anything can be established in general," opines a
modern naturopathic physician.[30]

The world shook Reichenbach's hand as a scientific industri-
alist who developed paraffin and creosote, but refused to shake
his hand as an investigator of Od: "Od," said the world, "does
not exist, and the bio-magnetism (mesmerism) based on it is
nothing more than prettily disguised hypnotism!"

Hypnosis—Is a Fluid Involved?

Firstly, a large number of distinguished researchers still take the
view, even today, that reciprocal action is involved. Hypnotism
more or less involves a fluid; and the fluid is the primary agent,
but is accompanied by fixation and verbal suggestion. I will mention here only the names Emile Boirac (1851–1917),[31] Dr. Erich
Kindborg,[32] formerly a general practitioner in Breslau, Dr. Sidney
Alrutz,[33] sometime lecturer at the University of Upsala. Dr.

---

[29]Reichenbach, Dr. Karl, *Odisch-magnetische Briefe* [Letters on Od and Magnetism] The
"Panopticum Medicum" collection] (Ulm/Donau: Karl F. Haug Verlag).
[30]Riedlin, Gustav, *Grundsachen der Krankheiten und Wahre Heilmitte* [The Fundamental
Causes of Diseases and their True Remedies] (Lorch h i.W: 1922), p. 176.
[31]Oirac, Emile, *Le Psychologie inconnue* [Unknown Psychology] (Paris, 1908).
[32]Kindborg, Dr. Erich, "Das Problem des Hypnotismus" [The Problem of Hypnotism],
Okkulte Welt, 1922, Nr. 101–102).
[33]Alrutz, Sidney, *Neue Strahlen des menschlichen Organismus: Ein Beitrag zum Problem der
Hypnose* (Stuttgart, 1924).

Walther VOELLER believes that now, after many years' research in the field of organo-electricity, that he has found the cause of hypnosis in this force."[8]

BIOMAGNETISM NOT BASED ON SUGGESTION

Secondly: we have four striking pieces of evidence that biomagnetism is based not on suggestion but on the transfer of a fluid. Medical specialist Dr. Ludwig LASZKY (Vienna) presented to Dr. Moritz BENEDIKT (died 1920) of the University of Vienna, "a laundress whose low intelligence completely ruled out any possibility that she knew about the crossover of the cerebral nerves" (indeed, some very well-educated individuals are ignorant of it). "I placed myself *behind* her and held my palm over the left side of the top of her head *without touching her at all*; whereupon she stuck her right leg out horizontally. When I held my palm over the right side of the top of her head, her left leg flew horizontally into the air. After this came the *experimentum crucis* (the acid test): Then, in the presence of the professor, I performed the countersuggestion test."

"After the left leg had executed its movement, I said, 'That was most interesting, we will do it once more.' But *surreptitiously* I changed the hand and side of the head *while standing behind her*, upon which her *other* leg responded right away. I believe there is no more striking evidence for the fact that magnetism has nothing to do with suggestion but is purely material."[34]

Dr. Josef GRATZINGER (died 1924), a mesmerist also resident in Vienna, said in 1922: "One of my patients came in my consultation hour and brought a dog with her which was suffering from a fairly extensive rash. While I was treating his mistress, the animal lay at her feet, *shut its eyes* and, to begin with, be-

---

[8]See original footnote, page 2.
[34]LASZKY, Dr. L., "Die magnetischen Kräfte des Menschen und die Praxis des Heilmagnetismus" [Animal Magnetism in Humans and the Practice of Healing Magnetism], *Okkulte Welt*, 1922, No. 131, pp. 15–16.

haved quite peacefully. After a while, another lady who was present noticed that in perfect time with the passes I was making with my hands, tremors ran through the body of the dog. However, his mistress thought that he might be shivering cold. Therefore I asked her to bring the dog when she came again, which she did next day. The dog lay down exactly as before and both I and several others who were present could observe that it lay still for a full five minutes and did not shiver in the slightest. When we were all agreed on this point, *I positioned myself behind the dog in such a way that it was impossible for it to detect my purpose,* and I made a few passes in its direction *at a distance of about a metre* and the tremors began straight away—now stronger, now weaker, according to how I made the passes. I also succeeded in producing at will tremors in its head, tail, paws, and even through its whole body. Some weeks later I had to visit a man suffering from encephalitis (brain fever), and again I had the opportunity to create by *distant passes* the most violent tremors in various parts of the body of a dog lying beside the patient's bed *with its eyes shut.* With this animal, too, I repeated the experiment *on different days* and *always with the same result. . . .* Thus it seems to have been demonstrated beyond doubt at last, by these animal experiments, that a real influence is exercised on the nervous system of the patient during our treatments, and suggestion does not have the lion's share in our results."[35]

In the summer of 1849, LAFONTAINE mesmerized in Livorno two out of six lizards and kept all of them without food. The non-mesmerized died after 9, 11, 13 and 18 days; the mesmerized lived for 42 and 75 days respectively, and then perished by accident."[36] Therefore the ones that were "handled" must have been kept alive by a subtle substance (a fluid!)

There are many examples of the growth of plants being "forced" by a supply of water that has been magnetized by pro-

[35]GRATZINGER, Dr. Joseph, *Das magnetische Heilverfahren: Handbuch für Ärzte und Laien* [Magnetic Healing: A Handbook for Doctors and Lay People] (Published privately by the author: Vienna, 1922), pp. 47–48.
[36]LAFONTAINE, pp. 328–329; SCHRÖDTER, *Grenzwissenschaftliche Versuche für jedermann* [Parapsychological Experiments for All] (Freiburg, i.B.: Bauer Verlag, 1959).

jecting rays on it or making passes over it with the hands. And this has been done in scientifically controlled conditions![37]

BIOMAGNETISM—AN ESTABLISHED FACT

Thus whoever looks with an open mind for evidence of the existence of a subtle emanation will find it here. Additional arguments in favor of it will be found in the works of LASZKY and GRATZINGER; also in my book, *Grenzwissenschaftliche Versuche*. Whoever feels "the rivers of living water" flowing "out of his belly" (Jno. 7:38), the *aqua vitae* of the physiological alchemist, "our heavenly water that does not wet the hands and is no ordinary water," will not need such evidence.

To those, however, who are dismissive on *a priori* grounds, the words of Arthur SCHOPENHAUER (1788–1860) still apply: "Whoever doubts the facts of animal magnetism (and of clairvoyance) nowadays ought to be called not sceptical but ignorant."[38]

MORE TO BIOMAGNETISM THAN PEOPLE THINK

The clinician and surgeon, Prof. Johann Nepomuk VON NUSSBAUM (1829–1890), privy councilor and Director-General of the Bavar-

---

[37]BERTRAM, Dr. Carl, "Der Mensch als Sender" [Human Transmitters], *Prana-Bücher*, No. 1 p. 51f; GOGOL, Gustav, "Die wohltätigen Einwirkungen des Magnetismus auf Pflanzen" ["The Beneficial Effects of Magnetism on Plants"] Z. *Heilmag-netismus*, 1928, 12 [March]: 96) Halle a.d.S; GROBE-WUTISCHKY, Arthur, *Fakirwunder und moderne Wissenschaft* [Fakir Miracles and Modern Science] (Berlin: Pankow, 1923), p. 69; LAFONTAINE, 340 f; OHLHAVER, Heinrich, *Die Toten leben* (Hamburg, 1916) p. 77; DU PREL, Baron Carl, "Die Pflanzen und der Magnetismus" ["Animal Magnetism and Plants"], *Über Land und Meer*, No. 46, 1885–1886); DU PREL, Baron Carl, "Pflanzenmystik, Teil 1, Das Magnetisieren von Pflanzen" ["Plant Mysticism, Part 1: The Magnetic Treatment of Plants"], *Sphinx* (1889), January issue, 17 f.; DU PREL, "Forciertes Pflanzenwachstum" ["Forced Plant Growth"] *Sphinx* (1889), March issue: 145 f.; WEDER, Wilhelm, *Magnetotherapie: Der Lebensmagnetismus als Heilmittel* (Nuremberg, 1892), p. 53 f.
[38]SCHOPENHAUER, Arthur, *Parerga and Paralipomena*. I; 261.

ian Army Medical Services, had this to say, among other things, in a book written for the general public:

After only a few minutes one can achieve a quite conspicuous, even astonishing result. The virtue of most ointments lies only in the rubbing. The hand of a certain person is often particularly comforting to someone who is nervous. Without doubt magnetic and electrical components come into play here. It cannot be denied that for each of us contact with some individual is more pleasant than with others, and in general the touch of a stranger's hand is unsettling. The hand of its loving mother has a clearly soothing effect on the forehead of a sick child. For that reason we certainly dare not deny what we cannot explain today."[39]

More recently, a similar conclusion has been reached by Dr. Luisa Hösli of Zürich, in the light of the successes of spiritual healing: "There are many cases in which every medical treatment fails and the doctor must yield to the inexplicable. This is especially true of those results of spiritual healing that have no rational explanation . . ."[40]

Someone dressed in uniform and as big as a wardrobe enters a room and sits down; yet, in spite of his size and show, one immediately feels there is nothing in him. Conversely, an individual who looks like a nonentity can have such a powerful emanation that one, as it were, instantaneously feels the resonance of their "room-filling" radiation striking one's skin.[41]

On walking into a dark room, we can sense by its atmosphere whether anyone is there or not.[42]

In order to detect diseases in others, Carl HUTER (1861–1912) systematically heightened in himself this "scenting faculty," which

[39]VON NUSSBAUM, J.N., *Die Hausaptoheke* [The Medicine Chest], (Munich, n.d.), p. 97.
[40]HÖSLI, Dr. Luisa, "Irrationales aus der Welt des Arztes" ["Irrational Happenings from the Doctor's World"], *Neue Wiss.* (1935), 2. Aug./Sept./Oct.: 55.
[41]SCHRÖDTER, Willy, "Alchemi" [Alchemy], *Der Blick* (1957), 5/6: [footnote].
[42]DRESSER, Horatio W., *Methoden und Probleme der geistigen Heilbehandlung* [The Methods and Problems of Spiritual Healing] (Leipzig, 1902), p. 40.

slumbers in embryonic form in those who are not comp⌐ thick-skinned."[43]

LEOPOLD, the attendant of the Viennese mesmerist Rudolf THETTER, confessed after about two months that he had imagined the whole thing was a swindle when he took the job, but he had now changed his mind. The headaches from which for twenty years he had suffered every day from morning until two o'clock in the afternoon, had been banished simply by the air in the treatment room. He came to the conclusion that everything must be done by the "medicinal air." THETTER commented, "The room itself where mesmerism is performed contains magnetic forces."[44] This remark reminds one of something MEYRINK said: "The atmosphere had become so magnetically stifling, that when I inhaled I felt I was being throttled by invisible hands."[45]

BIOMAGNETIC DIAGNOSIS

"In May 1926 a sensational action was brought in the district court in Warsaw against one of the most honored and popular Polish academics, Dr. Oskar WOJNOWSKI, accusing him of the illegal practice of medicine. For a long time this learned man has been accepted as a kind of naturopath and miracle worker. He has specialized in herbalism, and has made a professional study of it in India. When making a diagnosis, all he does is to lay his hand on the sufferer's body. Dr. WOJNOWSKI claims to be able to identify most organic diseases by this method. He was awarded his Ph.D. in Heidelberg."[46]

Diagnosis by the laying on of hands is by no means as new or unique as the above press cutting might lead one to believe. Rather, it belongs to the store of experience of every professional "handler" of vital energy, where mesmeric diagnosis and therapy

---

[43]HUTER, Carl, Sämtliche Schriften [Collected Works] (Althofnaß bei Breslau).

[44]THETTER, pp. 109–110, 118; NIELSEN, sub. 93; p. 151 f.

[45]MEYRINK, Gustav, Der weiße Dominikaner [The White Dominican] (Leipzig-Munich, Berlin-Vienna, 1921), p. 259.

[46]Diagnose durch die Hand [Manual Diagnosis] (Frankfurt, 1926, May 13, first edition).

are part and parcel of one another. Thus the circling and stroking hand—to use the *immanist* BENEDIKT's technical term—or the person who causes his or her emanation to flow into someone else, feels during the *immanizing* process: this is where the patient is suffering, this is where the source of the pain is in the *immanized* individual. Whatever the disease, the *immanism* evokes a specific and unambiguous sensation in the healer."[47] What is more, The "unconscious divine" steps in.

If the healer stills his or her understanding and will when approaching a sick person, the "Id" or the "unconscious divine"—as the Viennese mesmerist, engineer Rudolf THETTER (1882–1957)—so graphically describes it—takes over. In such a state of "higher awareness"—not, we hasten to add, a damping down of consciousness (*abaissement du niveau mental*)—the arms and hands are guided with an assured authority which permits no resistance to the execution of "masterly" magnetic passes in comparison to passes used when the mind is in its normal waking state.[48]

SPRAWLING POSTURES

While we are on the subject, a discovery of my own deserves a brief mention. The human body, directed by entelechy (the "Archeus" of PARACELSUS) adopts during sleep certain sprawling postures (Indian asanas), which obviously have a compensatory purpose. One hand rests on the suffering or weakened ("odically deficient") place, as the case may be, while the other draws strength from a dissimilar ("odically over-full") place.[49]

---

[47]THETTER, pp. 109–110, 118; NIELSEN: sub. 93; p. 151 f.
[48]THETTER, pp. 107–108.
[49]SCHRÖDTER, Willy, "Rekelposen: Der Schlaf als Lehrmeister" [Sprawling Postures: Sleep as a Teacher] *Natur und Kultur* (1956), 3 [July]; "Nochmals Rekelposen" [More about Sprawling Postures] *op. cit.* (1959), 3 [July].

THE RANGE OF "DISTANT PASSES"

It is now time to say a little about the *range* of "negative passes," "passes in the air," or "hovering hand-holds" (Dr. BOENISCH). GRATZINGER made passes about a meter away over the dog. The Copenhagen miracle-worker, Dorothea IVERSEN (born 1899) "places any of the female patients from her over-crowded waiting room with her face to the wall, places two men as catchers behind the patient, extends her hands from the opposite side of the room and when she draws her hands back slightly the subject always falls backwards.[50] This test for impressionability is called the "Moutin reflex" for Dr. Lucien MOUTIN (1856–1919).[51] Thus "the miracle worker of the Taubenweg" was able to exert the influence over a room of 6–8 meters; a fair distance! But short in comparison with the odic *actio in distans* (action at a distance) of a certain Philipp Walburg KRAMER (1815–1899) who declared, "With a few passes I have had an overwhelming effect at a distance of thirty paces in an open space on a highly sensitive person." [52] Indeed REICHENBACH himself says, "I have a very sensitive subject *on whom the effect of my hands when I was making passes, did not peter out at a distance of 40 metres,* which was as far as I could measure after clearing a straight line through my room."[53]

VON TUCHER wrote to THOLUCK: "He (Hauser) described the effect of hands held out toward him without his knowing it as like a draught or breath. DAUMER (1800–1875) could sense a hand pointed at his back without his knowledge at a *distance of 250 paces,* and the rapport—if we may call it that—was most intense when the hand was continuously rotated."[54]

---

[50]MEYER, Hans, "Sie pustet sich telefonisch gesund!" [She Blows Down the Telephone and Makes You Well!], *Constanze* (1949), a September number: 4–5); P.H.M., "Wunderfrau" heilt Krankheiten durch das Telephone ["'Wonder-woman' Cures Diseases by Phone"], *Wochenend* (1949), 11 [March 18]: 4–5).

[51]MOUTIN, Dr. Lucien, *Le diagnostic de la suggestibilité* [The diagnosis of suggestibility] (Paris, 1896).

[52]KRAMER, Phil. W., *Der Heilmagnetismus* [Mesmerism] (Leipzig, 1907), p. 44: Lorch I. W., 1931, p. 55.

[53]V. REICHENBACH, Baron Karl, *Odisch-magnetische Briefe* [Letters on Od and Magnetism] (Stuttgart and Tübingen, 1852; Ulm./Donau: Karl F. Haug Verlag, 1955), p. 165.

[54]M. W. Sphinx, 346 (Daumer's data edited by author).

TREATMENT TIME

The time required for the influence to make itself felt appears to be relatively short, and it is probably safe to assume that in optimal cases the "twinkling of an eye" (including an "evil eye") is enough, given an extremely "psycho-inactive" test subject and an experimenter who is supercharged with Od. Take, for example, the "growth waves" discovered in the 1930s by the Bavarian civil engineer Fritz HILDEBRAND (Berlin-Zehlendorf). These had a length of 10 through 30 cm., and seeds exposed to them for only 15 seconds underwent changes of such a kind that they produced plants much bigger than untreated ones and gave a yield of 100 percent as against the usual 40 percent.[55] Whereas HILDEBRAND needed a complicated electrical apparatus to broadcast his "growth waves," Surgeon-General Alexander HEERMANN, M.D. (1863–1946) produced them by the simplest means, and he too says that "it is noteworthy that the *irradiation time* is always very short, even for fodder, and ranges between a few seconds and one minute."[56]

OD IS NOT BIO-ELECTRICITY!

As regards HILDEBRAND'S wave generator, it should be pointed out that *Od is not the electricity of the body!* Back in 1805, an attempt was made to explain it away by Jacques Henri Désiré PÉTETIN (1744–1808), who called it "vital electricity" or "animal electricity."[57] Also electrical engineer E. K. MÜLLER (Kilchberg), director of the "Salus" in Zürich, saw at first in an "emanation of the living human body," which he called "Anthropoflux," "a special form of electricity," or "an energy resembling electricity"; however, in 1932, he announced that he had succeeded (using

[55]STÖLTING, Walter, "Sie können wachsen—wie Sie wollen!" ["You Can Grow Things How You Want Them"], *Scherls Magazin* (1930), 10 [Oct.]: 1025–1028.
[56]HEERMANN, Dr. Alexander, *Neues von Strahlen, Strömen und Wellen* [The Latest on Rays, Currents and Waves] (Bad Aussee, 1935), p. 9.
[57]SCHROEDER, H. E. Paul, *Geschichte des Lebensmagnetismus und des Hypnotismus* [A History of Animal Magnetism and Hypnotism] (Leipzig, 1889), p. 582; PÉTETIN, J. H. D., *Electricité animale* [Animal Electricity] (Lyon, 1805).

electrical apparatus!) in obtaining the objective evidence that "the emanation is not of an electrical nature!"[58]

PHYSICS AND BODY RADIATION

"When giving an effective treatment, the mesmerist feels a loss of vital energy, which has nothing whatever to do with the muscular force employed."[59] GRUNEWALD demonstrated this in the years 1917–1920 by his "ballistic measurement method" applied to 115 therapeutic treatments given by Peter JOHANNSEN. When he arranged for the latter to send a concealed treatment through the air, the magnetic intensity of the test subject increased "quite strangely" after a quarter of an hour! Which "clearly" proved that the phenomenon was solely magnetic and not electrical.[60]

REDISCOVERY OF OD

As a matter of fact, REICHENBACH's Od has been repeatedly rediscovered. For example, in 1903 it reappeared under the guise of the "N(ancy)-rays" of the physicist René-Prosper BLONDLOT (1849–1930), professor at the University of Nancy. His academic colleague, the physician, physiologist, and neurologist, Dr. Pierre Marie Augustin CHARPENTIER (1852–1916) took part in the planning of his research.[61]

---

[58]Müller, E. K., *Objektiver, elektrischer Nachweis der Existenz einer "Emanation" des lebenden menschlichen Körpers* [Objective Electrical Evidence of the Existence of an Emanation from the Living Human Body] (Basel, 1932), p. 32.
[59]BUTTENSTEDT, Carl, *Die Übertragung der Nervenkraft* [The Transfer of Nerve Force] (Rüdersdorf bei Berlin, n.d., ca. 1895), p. 121.
[60]GRATZINGER, 54 f.; according to Dr. Alfred GRADENWITZ, "Magnetische Menschen" [Magnetic People], in *Neues Wiener Journal* of August 11, 1921; GRUNEWALD, Fritz, *Ferromagnetische Erscheinungen am Menschen* [Ferromagnetic Phenomena in Humans] (Leipzig, 1922).
[61]SCHNEIDER, Emil, *Der animale Magnetismus* [Animal Magnetism] (Zürich, 1950), p. 443–444; FEERHOW, Friedrich (1888–1921), *N-Strahlen und Od: Ein Beitrag zum Problem der Radioaktivität der Menschen* [N-Rays and Od: A Contribution to the Study of Radioactivity in Humans] (Leipzig, 1912); Also: *Eine neue Naturkraft oder eine Kette von Täuschungen?" Reichenbachs Od und seine Nachentdeckungen* [A New Force of Nature or a Series of Deceptions?: Reichenbach's Od and Its Rediscoveries] (Leipzig, 1914); GEFFKEN, Dr. Heinrich, *Neues über N-Strahlen* (Diessen).

As we have seen, the *exposure time* may be quite short; especially if the distance between the two individuals is small. The "percipient" is so to speak "overshadowed" (Acts 5:15) and "the influence spreads from one body to the other" (THETTER). Distance is obliterated in the case of *positive passes*, that is to say, in the case of passes making direct contact with the subject—and generally speaking in all manipulations through the clothes or with skin contact; which a recent author calls *hand-laying*, implying that healing by the laying on of hands was the original mode of cure. Anyhow, the ancient Romans had two words for contact: *contactus* for the salubrious kind and *contagio* for the noxious. The distance is greater in "breathing upon" the subject, or aspiration, and also in "breathing into," or insufflation (which was formerly used *in extremis* as recorded in the Bible (2 Kings 4:34). But if the space between the two individuals is reduced without any reduction in the exposure time—as normally happens in encounters!—the influence will be noticeably increased.

OD-CARRIERS AND AMULETS

We can equate with manipulation or mesmerism by touch, the application, putting on, or wearing of "odically impregnated" objects ("substitutes"). Textiles and paper, among other things, are readily charged with Od. Carriers made of these materials throw a new light on the old belief in amulets, insofar as these *hamâle* (Arabic for "pendant") are made of these substances. *By way of reminder:* whereas the *amulet* possesses only a defensive (or protective) character, the talisman (Arabic: *telsamân* = magical diagram; from the Greek, *telesma* = payment) has a commanding force, and has been employed in every time and place as a bringer of good fortune.[62] Along these lines we can explain the ef-

---

[62]LAARSS, R. H. (Dr. Richard Hummel; 1870–1948), *Das Buch der Amulette und Talismane* [The Book of Amulets and Talismans] (Leipzig, 1919, 1932); WINCKELMANN, Joachim, *Das Geheimnis der Talismane und Amulette* [The Secret of Talismans and Amulets] (Freiburg, i. Br., 1955); VILLIERS, Elizabeth and PACHINGER, A. M., *Amulette und Talismane und andere geheime Dinge* [Amulets and Talismans and Other Esoterica] (Munich, 1927).

fect of the metallic materials used in *metallotherapy* (and in acupuncture)—apart from the power of suggestion, which must not be overlooked, of course—also the way in which vegetable materials affect us by their smell, radioactivity, and mitogenic radiations.

Bruno GRÖNING (1906–1959) used to press into the hands of those who had come for healing pellets he had rolled from the silver-paper or tinfoil linings of cigarette packets. Nowadays [1960] the paper-thin tinfoil is fast being replaced by the cheaper aluminium foil. Each of these metals, however, has special properties, and GRÖNING has conatively hit on something useful. Foil made of genuine tin is a good accumulator and storer of electricity of all kinds and also, it should be noted, of Od. To appreciate this, one has only to think of the coating of a Leyden jar, of the storage of tea in China in small containers of tinfoil[63] and of homeopathic high potencies being kept in the USA in medicinal bottles covered with tinfoil![64] Sheets of aluminium foil, used by Dr. Kurt TRAMPLER (Gräfelfing bei Munich) as receiving aerials,[65] are activated by *earth rays*, blacken photographic plates, and so serve as indicators of tellurian emanations.[66]

RELICS

At the same time, light is thrown on the source of the worldwide, persistent faith in relics; which has been taken so far that *copies* of (presumed genuine) relics are touched in order to get something from them (leaving one to wonder if it is not the touchers who are "touched"!).

---

[63]YUTANG, Lin, *Weisheit des lächelnden Lebens* [The Wisdom of the Smiling Life] (Stuttgart-Berlin, 1938), p. 254.

[64]SURYA, G. W, "Homöopathie, Isopathie, BiochemieIatrochemiund Elektrohomöopathie" [Homeopathy, Isopathy, Biochemistry, Iatrochemistry and Electrohomeopathy, Vol. VIII of the collection, *Okk. Med.* (1923), p. 37 f.

[65]TRAMPLER, Kurt, *Gesundung durch den Geist* [Spiritual Healing] (Munich-Planegg, 1953).

[66]DOBLER, Dr. Paul, *Physikalischer und photographischer Nachweis der Erdstrahlen* (Physical and Photographic Evidence of Earth Rays] 1934; WINCKELMANN, Joach. "Ein Beitrag für Strahlenforscher" [A Contribution to Radiation Research], *Neue Wiss.* (1956), 4 f.

"ANEMIC" PEARLS

Also to the point here is the empirical finding that pearls lose their luster when their wearer's vital energy is low, and regain their original beauty when transferred to a completely healthy ("supercharged") individual. For the cure of "anemia in pearls" Oriental potentates employed highly-endowed "pearl wearers." What is more, a regular pearl hospital has recently been opened in Chicago.[67]

BOLTZIANISM

The first-named category of *Od-carriers* (i.e., fabrics) sheds light on Boltzianism, named for the Swedish pastor, Friedrich August BOLTZIUS (1836–1910), in which—as in early Christian times (Matt. 14:36, Luke 8:44, Acts 19:12)—pieces of clothing belonging to the "dispensers of healing" are worn by patients.

TELEPATHY

The existence of telepathy appears to have been broadly verified by the quantitative-statistical research methods employed at Duke University since 1930, in collaboration with animal psychologist Prof. McDOUGALL (1875–1938), by Prof. Joseph Banks RHINE (born 1895), and also by the series of scientific tests carried out by Prof. Hans BENDER (born 1907), director of the Institute for Frontier Research into Psychology and Mental Hygiene in Freiburg i.Br.[68]

---

[67]SCHRÖDTER, Willy, "Lithotherapie" [Stone Therapy], Erfahr.Hk. (1957), 5 [May]: 221 f.; FÜHNER, H., *Lithotherapie* (Ulm/Donau: Karl F. Haug Verlag, 1955).

[68]GERSTER, Dr. G., *Eine Stunde mit* . . . [Aus der Werkstatt des Wissens I (Ullstein-Buch Nr. 73)] [An hour with . . . [From the workshop of knowledge I (Leipzig, 1940), pp. 67, 228; FRITSCHE, Dr. Herb, *Tierseele und Schöpfungsgeheimnis* [Animal Souls and the Secret of Creation] (Leipzig, 1940), pp. 67, 228; RHINE, J. B., *The Reach of the Mind* (New York, 1947); *New World of the Mind* (New York, 1954); RINGGER, Dr. Peter, *Parapsychologie. Die Wissenschaft des Okkulten* [Parapsychology: The Science of the Occult] (Zürich, 1957), p. 33.

But even if there were no theoretical arguments or scientific evidence in favor of "brain waves," their existence would be rendered probable by everyday observations.

As far as theory is concerned, the physical chemist Dr. Paul VAGELER (Addis Ababa) held the view that: "Speaking as a physicist, the existence of electromagnetic "brain waves" as a by-product of the atomic layering in the brain and resonance in other, receptive brains, and therefore the existence of thought projection, is about as self-evident as twice two is four. If one knew of no examples of thought transference, one would be compelled to look for them. For they simply must exist from the point of view of physics, given the appropriate conditions, the strength of the sender, and the vacancy of mind of the receiver."[69]

In December 1929 the provincial court in Leitmeritz (Czechoslovakia) was the scene of a case brought against the telepathist and clairvoyant, Erik Jan HANUSSEN (Herschmann STEINSCHNEIDER; 1889-1933). The district attorney asked the expert witness, Prof. Oskar FISCHER, psychiatrist, of the University of Prague: "Wouldn't you agree that you are sowing the seeds of superstition among the populace with your views?" To which the expert responded: "In reply to your question I have to say to you that it is a much greater superstition to deny the existence of telepathy and clairvoyance."[70] Prestigious and high-ranking witnesses appeared for the defense during this trial which ran for weeks. In court, the accused was so accurate in answering the problems put to him that, in finding him not guilty, the tribunal presided over by judge Robert SCHALECK, certified that, "In the opinion of the court, the defendant does indeed possess mysterious mental powers, since their effect has been confirmed by numerous credible witnesses."

On the basis of compelling theoretical considerations and empirical observations, the French philosopher, Henri BERGSON (1859–1941)—one of the "immortals" of the Académie française —once declared: "*I am as much compelled* to believe in telepathy as

[69]VON KLINCKOWSTROEM, Count Karl, *Yogi-Künste* [Yogic Arts], *Collection of Die okk. Welt.* (1922), No. 99, p. 31.
[70]HERMANN, Dr. H., "Albert Einstein über Parapsychologie" ["Albert Einstein on Parapsychology"], *Neue Wiss.* (1955), 8–9 [August/September]: 280.

to believe that the defeat of the 'invincible armada' (August 7 and 8, 1588) was an actual event."

PHYSICAL EVIDENCE OF BRAIN-WAVE EMISSION

In 1926 a work appeared in German from the pen of Dr. Ferdinando CAZZAMALLI (died 1958), at that time professor of neurology in the University of Mailand, according to which he had demonstrated by means of a radio set the "broadcasting of 'brain waves' during telepathic phenomena."[71]

Prof. CRILE (Cleveland, OH) later photographed the weak radiation of human brain tissue, which varies in luminosity according to the time of year. This had been demonstrated long before by Dr. Max DE CRINIS of the Graz University hospital. Prof. Hans BERGER (1873–1941), director from 1919 through 1938 of the University Mental Hospital in Jena, developed the electroencephalogram in 1924 and publicly unveiled it in 1929.

Building on the work of RHINE, the United States army has recently conducted experiments with "brain waves" involving "the sending of messages over great distances (telepathy) as well as "acting on objects" (psychokinesis). Its scientists "regard it as probable that brain waves are akin to radar."[72]

TELEPATHY DEPENDS ON UNDULATORY WAVES

The concept that telepathy depends on waves or rays can be traced from Abu Jussuf Jacub Ebn Eshalk ALKINDI (ca. 750) until we come to VÖLGYESI in modern times. The court astrologer of the Caliph Abu, Giafur AL-MANSUR (754–775) proposed in *De Imaginibus* that the so-called *actio in distans* [action at a distance] happened *per*

---

[71]CAZZAMALLI, Ferdinando, "Ausstrahlung von 'Gehirnewellen' bei telepsychischen Phänomenen" ["The Radiation of 'Brain Waves' in Telepsychic Phenomena"] Z. *Parapsychol.* (1926), February and March issue.

[72]"Gehirnwellen-Experimente" [Brain-Wave Experiments], *Die andere Welt* (1959), 2 [February] 43; taken from *Psykisk Forum* [Copenhagen], December 1958, which quoted in turn from an article in the Herald Tribune.

certos radios [by means of certain rays].[73] He was thinking no doubt of certain "dastardly deeds" performed by visualization (purposeful fantasy), similar to those later recorded by his famous compatriot AVICENNA (Abu Ali al-Hussein IBN SINA; 979–1036): some individuals are able from a distance to make a camel fall over together with its rider. This "art" is still practiced today.

Eira HELLBERG (of Stockholm) watched while an Englishman—who had resided in India for many years and had learned much—made a girl fall off her bicycle.[74] Conversely, STRINDBERG witnessed how a "witch"—also acting from a distance—prevented a woman from mounting her bicycle. The woman was unable to do so until her "ill-wisher" turned her head and looked away, hissing, "Up on it with you!"[75] Objective mechanical evidence has been produced that telepathy depends on undulatory waves, as I have established elsewhere.[36] Here are three more cases:

1. Professor St. at the psychology seminar in the University of B. demonstrated a "thought-ticker" as long ago as 1910. Using the requisite concentration, a test subject caused the little apparatus to ring at the other end of the room.[76]

2. When an impulse of the will is sent into a hand in a plaster cast, it has the effect of producing flashes of light in a glass vacuum tube some 3–4 m. away if one pole of the tube is connected to a TESLA current.[77]

3. Several years ago, in the Physiology Department of the University of Vienna, in several hundred trials, the ideation of clenching the fist was made audible as a creaking and crackling coming from several loudspeakers and amplifiers.[78]

---

[73]LUDWIG, Dr. Aug. Frdr., *Geschichte der okkulten Forschung* [A History of Occult Research] (Pfullingen i.W., 1922), I, p. 57.

[74]HELLBERG, Eira, *Telepathie: Okkulte Kräfte* [Telepathy: Occult Forces] (Prien/Obb., 1922), p. 153.

[75]STRINDBERG, August, *Ein drittes Blaubuch* [A Third Bluebook] (Munich, 1921), p. 1044.

[36] See earlier footnote, p. 14.

[76]ZEISS, Max, "Lautsprechende Gedankenübertragung" ["Thought Transference as a Public Address System"], *Zbl. Okk.* (1925), 321.

[77]KRAUSE, Prof., "Die neuesten wiss. Experimentierergebnisse der biomagnetische Heilweisse" ["The Latest Scientific Experimental Results Concerning Biomagnetic Treatment"], *Z. Heilmagnetismus* (1930), August issue: 58 f.

[78]GERSTER, sub. 64, p. 196.

"This proves that our will and the activity of the cerebrospinal system are enough to cause emission to the outside of a detectable radiation."[77] In my own opinion, the "cerebrospinal radiation"—which seems to be clearly demonstrated here—is only the *effectus* (operation) in the *physis* (in nature) of what is being thought; its cause, I believe, is in the transphysis!

Evidence that *thoughts are things* is always available to anyone prepared to construct a simple piece of apparatus. This point will be taken up later on under the heading "Chevreuil's pendulum experiments," but first I want to let everyday telepathic experiences speak for themselves.

An appropriate transition to our next investigation is the opinion expressed in 1938 by Dr. Franz (Ferenc) VÖLGYESI (born 1895), a Budapest-born medical hypnotist renowned throughout Europe: "What a host of mysteries still lies concealed under the *radiated influences* brought to bear by *telepathic means* by person on person, animal on animal, and person on animal (and vice versa); of which a very easily understood and precise illustration is the extraordinarily subtle, synchronized and tuned resonance of radio transmitters and receivers, which occurs in countless places at the same time, and in all directions (although not so long ago we scarcely ventured to think of such a thing).[79]

DISTANT TRANSMISSION FROM ANIMALS TO HUMANS

A good example of unwanted transmission of this sort is ailurophobia: cats are able, even when their presence is unknown, unseen, unheard, and unsmelled by a visitor, to produce more or less disagreeable sensations in the latter, possibly to the point where they become unbearable,[80] often when they are quite a way away![81]

---

[79]VÖLGYESI, Dr. Franz, *Menschen- und Tierhypnose* [Hypnotism in Humans and Animals] (Zürich and Leipzig, 1938), p. 29.
[80]CARUS, Carl Gustav, *Über Lebensmagnetismus und die magnetischen Wirkungen überhaupt* [Animal Magnetism and Magnetic Effects in General] (Basel, 1925), pp. 83, 115.
[81]KLUGE, Carl Al. Ferd., *Versuch einer Darstellung des animalischen Magnetismus als Heilmittel* [An Attempt to Present Animal Magnetism as a Means of Cure] (Berlin, 1815), p. 244, § 205.

So, for example, Joseph BONAPARTE (1786–1844), ex-king of Naples, later of Spain, was laid low for some hours at Saratoga Springs (New York) in 1825 on the occasion of a banquet hosted by Henry WOLTON. The villain of the piece was a tiny cat hiding under a sideboard. Joseph's big brother, Napoleon BONAPARTE (1769–1821) was also an ailurophobe but not the first to ascend the throne of France, for King Henri III (1574–1589) always passed out at the sight of a cat.

DISTANT TRANSMISSION FROM HUMANS TO ANIMALS

It is notorious that a domestic pet, especially a dog or cat, can be aware of its owner's return long before he or she arrives or is in range of the animal's sense of smell, that they can perceive the owner's death at a distance, can be summoned by them, and even (in extreme cases) be induced to perform certain actions. What our much-quoted author, Marie CORELLI narrates in her novel *A Romance of Two Worlds* (New York: F.M. Lupton, n.d., Ch. IX, p. 148) about a dog telepathically influenced by a man to perform certain actions: "This animal, commanded—or, I should say, brain-electrified by Heliobas, would fetch anything that was named to him through his master's force, provided it was light enough for him to carry," HELLBERG (who is also quoted more than once) reports as a fact (p. 153)!

"Thinking" or "talking" animals fall into this category.[82] The dog, for example, is the "delegated unconscious of its owner" (FRITSCHE). In fact, this is something that has a veterinary use. Queen Elizabeth II of England arranged for one of her horses, the favorite "Aureole," to be treated for neurosis by a certain Charles BROOK, who achieved a cure by close contact and encouragement. The telepathic component is obvious here. One newspaper reporter referred to the healer as a "quack" (from "quack-salver"—"quicksilver-salver"). The taunt was unjustified, because the so-called "quack" was 100 percent successful,

---

[82]FRITSCHE, Dr. Herbert, *Tierseele und Schöpfungsgeheimnis* [Animal Souls and the Secret of Creation] (Leipzig, 1940).

and the racehorse won 2,000 pounds sterling in prize money in the Derby![83]

TELEPATHY BETWEEN ANIMALS

This is evident in butterflies, ants, and termites. It occurs so regularly in the "white ant" that Maurice Polydore Marie Bernard MAETERLINCK (1862–1949) was inclined to see a single individual in the termite nest.[84] Eugène N. MARAIS (died 1937) spoke of a termitary and a composite animal.

This collective, which is often as high as 10 meters, somehow generates, by its telepathic communication, electric currents of such intensity that they are liable to interfere with shortwave reception in the neighborhood. It was for this reason, according to a press report, that firemen were employed to destroy a termitary near Lima. One could view the cellular commonwealth of our body machinery as a compound animal, too: "For there is not only telepathy from brain cells to brain center, but also telepathy between cells, as has already been alluded to by SCHLEICH. I recall, for example, an experimental inoculation of TB bacilli in the abdominal cavity of a guinea-pig, with the immediate result that, by telepathic command, leukocytes converged like security police from all parts of the body to arrest the intruders."[8]

DEFINITION OF THE TERM "TELEPATHY"

Before producing convincing proof from everyday life of the reality of telepathy, I believe it is in order to point out that to render this Greek-based technical term by the words thought transference is inaccurate. The true translation is "far-sensing"

---

[83]PRIUS: "Quacksalber Ihrer britischen Majestät" ["Quack by appointment to her Britannic Majesty"], *Volksstimme* (1953), 241, [October 17].

[84]LAKHOVSKY, pp. 242, 245; MAETERLINCK, Maurice, *La Vie des Termites* [The Life of Termites] (1926); MARAIS, Eugène N., *The Soul of the White Ant* (London, 1953).

[8]See earlier footnote, page 2.

(*tele* = "far," *pathein* = "to suffer, to sense"). And it is impor⟨ to note that most people experience (*pathein*) an indistinct, ⟨ scure, formless, sensitive resonance (prescience or inner certainty) in response to the feeling, thinking, and awareness of a second person some distance away, and that the translation of this impression into a clearly formulated idea occurs only in a minority of individuals (the abstract thinkers?). Finally, the conversion of reflected waves of emotion into symbolic or encoded, valid, clearcut pictures (clairvoyance in space) happens only in a few who possess eidetic imagery—as a divine gift or by heavenly decree?

There is nobody who has not had some such experience as the following:

1. Seeing a sleeper (adult or child) wake up when we fix our eyes on them;

2. Finding that on staring at the nape of the neck, or the occiput, of an acquaintance sitting several rows in front of us, and willing them to become aware of our presence, they grow restless, turning their head from side to side and then around to look at us.[85]

The nape (or back) of the neck, which externally is an indentation and internally is the place where the *medulla oblongata* goes through the occiput, plays an important part in occultism. It is the *Uls* of the ancient Egyptian magicians,[86] the *Lus* of the Jewish Kabbalists, the "divine mouth" in Indian Kriya Yoga, and the exit-point of a hypothetical subtle "meta-organism."[87] What is more, Professor of Zoology, Dr. Gustav JAEGER (1832–1917), recommended sniffing at the neck hairs of patients, and performing distant healing magnetism if their smell was disagreeable to the operator. "In the nape of the neck, in the region of the decussation of the nerves of the brain, the radiation is strongest and therefore most easily detected."[88]

---

[85]SCHRÖDTER, Willy, *Streifzug ins Ungewohnte* [A Voyage into the Unusual] (Freiburg i.Br., Germany, 1949), p. 63.
[86]KIESEWETTER, Carl, *Der Okkultismus des Altertums* [The Occultism of Antiquity] (Leipzig, 1896), pp. 276–277.
[87]RIJNBERK, G. A., *Les Métasciences biologiques* [The Biological Metasciences] (Paris, 1952), p. 12.
[88]JAEGER, Gustav, *Die Entdeckung der Seele* [The Discovery of the Soul] (Leipzig, 1880).

In the occiput, under the crown of the head, the pineal gland is housed, the rudimentary *parietal* or "third" eye *(Shivas)*. The Munich paleontologist and philosopher, Edgar DACQUÉ (1878–1945) writes in this connection in his *Urwelt, Sage und Menschheit* [The Primeval World, Myth, and Mankind] (1924): "Let us envisage the physical appearance of primitive humans. The epiphyseal eyes in particular were of a lower type. The epiphyseal eye has been the characteristic organ of every primitive age. It was definitely not an eye simply for seeing with; for the higher animals of those times, as later, possessed it in addition to their two well-developed normal eyes. Thus it can only be the organ of a sense that has been lost by modern animals and humans—the *pineal gland*, now overgrown by the cerebrum. If the cerebrum is the seat of the intellect, and has brought about an increasing loss of the demonic instinctive as it has grown more complex, so the complete withdrawal of the cerebrum and the full development of the underlying, but currently extinguished *parietal* organ, would entail the physical manifestation of that sense that usually leaves the field to the reflective intellect—the *naturally sighted.* The pineal gland or third eye was presumably the physically active, perceptive and executive organ of this lost, naturally sighted inner essence. Long before Renatus CARTESIUS (René DESCARTES; 1596–1650) did so, people had come to regard its shape as that of the soul. Thus on the pedestals on each side of the "Wolf's door" of Aachen cathedral, there are a wolf and a fir-cone or pine-cone made of brass. These are said to belong to the age of Charlemagne (768–814). Folk tradition has it that the pine-cone is the wolf's soul.[89]

The opinion that (unusually long) hair can pick up thought waves like an aerial has often been expressed. Thus in 1950 the surrealist Spanish painter, Salvador DALI (born 1904), who was then living in the USA, told a New York reporter that the twirled ends of his enormously long Tartar moustache were a sort of radar for him, with which he picked up ideas from the sea of thought. At about the same time, the French parapsychologist Dr. Henri ALAIN tried to prove scientifically that the hair is a telepathic receiver. Possibly the clerical tonsure was originally designed, among other things, to cut off mental influences from outside (Dr. LAFITTE).

---

[89]ZAUNERT, Dr. Paul, *Rheinland-Sagen* [Legends of the Rhine], vol. I (Jena, 1924), p. 71.

3. We can feel when someone creeps up on us from behind. "I could feel him coming along, skulking after me his eyes on my neck . . ." are the words put into the mouth of his character Molly Bloom concerning Boylan by James JOYCE (1882–1941) in *Ulysses* (p. 883).

4. Words are often said to be taken out of a person's mouth, as in: "That is just what I was going to say. . . ." "The one speaks what the other thinks."[90] In GOETHE (1749–1832) we have the example of two lovers playing charades during a stroll together and anticipating the solutions by some "subtle sense."

The ideal is wordless telepathic conversation like that between Madame GUYON (1648–1717) and her father confessor Père LACOMBE, of whom she said: "When Father Lacombe was admitted to hear my confession or to administer the sacraments to me, I could not talk to him without the same stillness arising in me as when I am in the presence of God. I gathered that God wished to teach me that humans can understand the language of angels even in this life. *Gradually I reached the stage where I was able to converse with Father Lacombe in complete silence.* And thus we comprehended each other in God in an inexpressible and heavenly way. *We spent hours in this deep silence, continually reading one another's thoughts, without being able to say a single word.*"[91]

Dr. Paul BRUNTON (New York) "hoped . . . to engage in *silent telepathic communication* with the century-old yellow sages in the Chinese hinterland and the Gobi desert."[92]

5. Anticipating the mail. Sitting in the office, one can tell the very moment when an eagerly awaited letter arrives at home. The American humorist Mark TWAIN (S.L. CLEMENS; 1835–1910) joined the two-year old "Society for Psychical Research" in London on October 4, 1884, because he had become a firm believer in telepathy or "mental telegraphy" owing to his frequent experiences of "postal prescience" as I call it.[93] Hans

---

[90]STERNEDER, Hans, *Sommer im Dorf* [Summer in the Village] (Leipzig, 1930), p. 164.
[91]HELLBERG, pp. 56–57.
[92]BRUNTON, Paul, *The Secret Path* (York Beach, ME: Weiser, 1985), p. 13.
[93]NIELSEN, Enno, *Das große Geheimnis usw.* [The Great Secret etc.] (Ebenhausen bei Munich, 1923), p. 243 f.

STERNEDER, known as the Austrian "apostle of miracles" and "peasant student," also has firsthand knowledge of the same phenomenon.[94]

6. The sad thoughts of one of a harmoniously linked couple will keep the other awake, even when nothing has been said about them, and no outward sign has been shown—not even tossing and turning in bed!

7. *Lupus in fabula* (the wolf in the fable, or "Speak of the Devil!"), or in the blunt speech of Rhenish Hessia: "Name the donkey and he'll come running." He will also come running if one merely thinks of him—perhaps even sooner, for the power does not reside in the words.[95] And why does one think of him? Because his intention to visit us runs ahead of him. "On the wings of the wind" as both Cornelius AGRIPPA[96] and the Tibetans[97] would put it. The numberless instances that have come to my attention over the years rule out "coincidence." The experience is universal. A Chinese proverb puts it in a nutshell: "Speak of Ts'ao Ts'ao and Ts'ao Ts'ao is sure to appear!"

8. Longing for certain individuals: this is much like the "wolf in the fable." Only here it is not because they intend coming that we think of our partner: they come because we want them to come. GOETHE says of himself: "In lovers the magnetic force is unusually powerful and even acts at a distance. I had sufficient proof of this when I was a young man, and on a lonely walk was overcome by a strong desire for a girl I was in love with and I thought about her for a very long time until she actually came to meet me. 'I felt restless in my little room,' she said, 'I could not help myself, I had to come here.'"[98]

---

[94]STERNEDER, pp. 162, 339.
[95]SCHRÖDTER, Willy, *Offenbarungen eines Magiers* [The Revelations of a Magician] (Warpke-Billerbeck, 1955), pp. 28, 30.
[96]AGRIPPA, vol. I, p. 65
[97]DAVID-NEEL, Alexandra, *Magic and Mystery in Tibet* (New York: University Books, 1958).
[98]ECKERMANN, Joh. Peter: *Gespräche mit Goethe* [Conversations with Goethe], October 7, 1827 (Weimar, 1837–1848); SCHRÖDTER, *Offenbarungen* [The Revelations], p. 29.

Conrad Ferdinand MEYER (1825–1898) witnessed how a merchant in Chur could summon his clerk telepathically whenever he wanted.[99]

MESSAGES FROM THE DYING

On a higher level, we shall now examine those cries for help picked up from a distance when someone dear to us is in danger ("SOS-telepathy") and also messages from the dying, both of which break in on our current train of thought with startling intensity (almost like some form of inspiration).

The indubitably authentic cases of *clocks stopping* when people die are legion. One has only to make a few inquiries in one's circle of friends to discover them![100] The reality of the phenomenon is so deeply ingrained in the mind of the people that Johann Gabriel SEIDL (1804–1875) took it as the theme of his ballad "Der tote Soldat" [The Dead Soldier] (based on an actual event in the 1870–1871 war):

There sits the mother weeping
With sobs that rise to heaven:
"He has been here to say farewell—
The clock stopped at eleven!"

What is more, this experience is widespread, since the Chinese, for example, avoid a room in which a clock has stopped for no apparent reason. The parapsychological explanation of this phenomenon is that the ticking of the clock is identified with his or her (often no longer perceptible) heartbeat by the dying person, and that at the moment the spirit is released from its physical ve-

---

[99]NIELSEN, nach "Ein Besuch bei C. F. Meyer" [after "A visit with C. F. Meyer"], September 17, 1892, p. 259.
[100]NIELSEN: *Geheimnis* [The Great Secret, etc.], p. 171; ROESERMUELLER, W. O., *Unsere "Toten" leben* [Our Dead Live](Nuremberg, 1958), p. 38; "Die Uhren bleiben stehen" [The Clocks Stop], Glaube u. Erkenntnis, 1953: 8–9 (Abensberg/Ndb.).

hicle (excarnation) it stops the timepiece *telekinetically* (Greek: "acting remotely").[101] In VOELLER'S opinion: "At the point of death there is a total organo-electric discharge from the body. An ensuing reciprocal effect on the objects concerned must be regarded as the cause of the said phenomenon."[102] A fairly extensive "organo-electric discharge from the body" seems to have been experienced by the Austrian attorney's wife who wrote to me on December 17, 1958 (among other things): "What is more, I am in poor health; although it is probably only (sic!) a state of exhaustion. I can't cope any longer and am at my wits' end. It is a curious fact that *all the clocks in my room, including any replacements I bring in, refuse to work.*" It is well known that the wristwatches—the handcuffs worn by the time-fixated people of the present era (sufferers from "angina temporis" in the expressive words of J. EICK and K. GAUGER)—of neurotic, epileptic and hysterical individuals[103] are unreliable and that, conversely, watches can influence their wearers when their metal cases press on the *acupuncture meridians*. However, the phenomenon is even more far-reaching than this: the "aura" or the "body's atmosphere" as KLUGE[104] terms it [KILNER'S "human atmosphere." *Tr.*], actually impregnates the room and its contents, as we shall see further on.

While we are on the subject of "clock stopping," it is worth bearing in mind the incredible statistical odds against such a probability calculated by foreign scientific societies.[105] "So-called *death-bed experiences* are among the most frequent and well-attested paranormal phenomena. The celebrated Swiss parapsychologist, Dr. Peter RINGGER (born 1923), has established that they are not confined to the familiar "warnings."[106]

---

[101]MEYRINK: *Dominikaner* [The White Dominican], p. 117.
[102]VOELLER, Dr. Walther, "Problem des siderischen Pendels, der Wünschelrute und der Tischrückens" [Problem of the sidereal pendulum, divining rod, and table turning], *Z. Heilmagnetismus* (1926), 9 [Dec.] 1968). Halle/S.
[103]JOYCE, vol. II, p. 339
[104]KLUGE, p. 251.
[105]VOGL, Dr. Carl, *Unsterblichkeit* [Immortality] (Dachau, 1917), p. 183 f.; DE FRÉMERY, H. N., *Telepathie* (Leipzig, 1905), 29 f.; *Proc. Soc. Psych. Res.* (London).
[106]RINGGER, sub 68, p. 103.

A TELEPATHIC NEWS AGENCY

We shall have to content ourselves with a very brief account of this, since it is not an everyday experience in the West. On the other hand, distant thought transmission is to the "Land of Snow" (Tibet) what wireless telegraphy is to us.[97] This finding of the French professor, expert on Tibetan Buddhism, and initiated "Lama-Dama," Alexandra DAVID-NEEL (born in 1878), has been confirmed by the Buddhist convert, Italian professor Giuseppe TUCCI, the French explorer in Tibet, Cécilie CORENTIN, and the French researcher, Aumary DE RIENCOURT.

"Since 1884 we have had more accurate information about a secret method of communication by which news is sent and received at a distance. This is called 'Hindostan,' and in Western Asia *Khabar*, the Arabic for news."[107]

Instances from the West are:

1. In 1937, the American author, SHERMAN, was in verified continuous telepathic contact with his friend, the polar aviator, Sir Hubert WILKINS, during the search made by the latter for the missing polar aviator, S. LEVANEWSKY: "From November 1937 to March 1938 sixty-eight highly successful cases of telepathic communications were achieved in this way."[108]

2. On eight evenings in the fall of 1949, the 23-year old Australian, Mrs. PIDDINGTON, located in the Tower of London, sent information supplied by prominent witnesses to her 31-year old husband Sidney in a BBC studio.[109] [In the case of the Pidding-

---

[97]See earlier footnote, p. 34.

[107]HELLBERG, p. 155 f.; KIESEWETTER, Karl, *Der Okkultismus des Altertums* [Occultism in Antiquity] (Leipzig, 1897), p. 218 f.; SCHRÖDTER, *Offenbarungen* [Revelations], pp. 12, 70; SCHRÖDTER, Willy: "Telepathischer Nachrichtendienst" [A Telepathic News Agency], *Neues Licht* (1951), 12 [Dez.], 228–229; and "Telepathischer Nachrichtendienst," *Neue Wiss.* (1956), 11–12, 336–353; Anonymous, "Menschliche Telephone" [Human Telephone], *Zbl. Okk.* (1942), February issue, 383.

[108]RINGGER, S., 34 f.; WILKINS and SHERMAN, *Thoughts through Space* (New York, 1942).

[109]VON BERGFELDE, Robert, "Okk. Sensation im Londoner Rundfunk" [Occult Sensation on London Radio], *Neues Zeitalter* (1949), 12 [October 28]: 4–5; SCHRÖDTER, Willy, "Telepathischer Nachrichtendienst" [A Telepathic News Agency], *Neues Licht* (1956), 6 [June], 110–111.

tons, without impugning anybody's good faith, it is probably wise to remember that theirs was a "live act" staged by a mixed news and entertainment medium (radio). This makes its true value more difficult to assess. *Translator's note*].

3. About the same time, the British boxing fraternity heard the sensational report that Don COCKELL, the 22-year old light-heavy-weight, had often, and from more than a hundred miles away, been kept free from fear and nervous tension in the ring by the telepathic intervention of S. W. J. MILLER, a psychophysiotherapist and lecturer at the "Institute of Life Science."[110]

Strictly speaking, Case 3 does not belong to this section, since it does not involve the telepathic transmission of information, which is our main interest here, but of beneficial calming and fortifying emotions.

HUMAN BEINGS AS ANTENNAE

Writers and poets are creators. They draw their creations from the ocean of thought, which pours over them and flows through them; and in words and writings addressed to others, they give solid shape to what they have picked up from afar. One or two of them, such as the seaman and popular writer Robert KRAFT,[111] have confessedly produced "their" works in a *trance* state, others, NIETZSCHE, for example, have written in an "ecstasy";[112] or, at any rate, "passive thinking" predominates in them.

In these bouts of elation, various prose writers or poets have given details or even names in their "creations" that have later turned out to be realities. Elsewhere I have cited ample instances.[113] *In this condition poetic activity approaches the Khabar!* But

[110]LEDERER, Kurt A. B., "Gedankenübertragung im Boxring" [Thought Transference in the Boxing Ring], *Okk. Welt* (1949), 3 [October 1]: 5); ANONYMOUS, "Gedankenübertragung im Boxring," *Hausfreund f. Stadt u. Land* (1949), 36 [September 31], 12.
[111]KRAFT, Robert, *Eine kurze Lebensbeschreibung von ihm selbst verfaßt* [A Brief Autobiography] (Dresden-Niedersedlitz: Die Augen der Sphinx. n.d.).
[112]KANKELEIT, Otto, *Das Unbewußte als Keimstätte des Bewußten* [The Unconscious as the Seedbed of the Conscious] (Munich/Basel, 1959), p. 27, 52–53.

if the poet can operate as a "receiver," it is also conceivable that, in certain circumstances, he or she may function as a "transmitter," and therefore that his or her "broadcast fantasies" (even if not printed and read!) could sow the seeds of good, and more probably of evil, deeds. At this point I am reminded of something said by Pablo PICASSO (born 1881) in his capacity as painter and graphic artist; who, in what strikes me as an often "unnatural" mode of representation, seems to be displaying the working of the unconscious, and thus should fit well into our theme. He said something to the effect that: "Even when I do not exhibit my pictures, but wrap and store them, their effect on third parties is not nullified."

On the subject of *random* thought transmission, Dr. Franz HARTMANN expressed the following opinion: "But people's thoughts also act on one another in an arbitrary fashion. We do not know from where our thoughts come (JOYCE [Ulysses I] says that one never knows whose thoughts one is chewing over), or where they go. (FEUCHTERSLEBEN said: 'Thoughts, emotions, attitudes, float unseen in the air; we breathe them in, assimilate them, and pass them on, without being fully aware of these processes.') They are like seed grains carried by the wind, which germinate wherever they find fertile soil; and from these seeds actions grow. *A lurid 'shocker' devised by a writer in one country, can lead by thought transmission to a tragic crime in another country*, and it is conceivable that a judge could sentence a criminal for a crime he himself had inspired by the unaware and unintentional projection of his own fantasy. This is unconscious 'black magic,' and we do not need to look very far for such occult phenomena. The world is full of examples, though we do not see them . . ."[114]

Whoever has witnessed how the *unexpressed* malicious thoughts of one individual are shortly afterward uttered by an *absent* second individual who is related to or in sympathetic con-

---

[113]SCHRÖDTER, Willy, *Abenteuer mit Gedanken* [Adventures with Thoughts] (Freiburg i. Br., Germany, 1954 p. 29 f.; and "Der Dichter—ein Seher" [The Poet—A Seer], *Neue Wiss.* (1958), 4 [Jan./Feb.]), 168 f.; and "Schöpfer oder Antenne? Vom dichterischen Wirken" [Creators or Pick-Up Aerials? On Writing Poetry], *Natur u. Kultur Folge* (1959), 1, 16f.

[114]HARTMANN, Dr. Franz, *Denkwürdige Erinnerungen* [Remarkable Memories] (Leipzig, ca. 1897), p. 145.

nection with the first, will not *a priori* reject the inference that a moment of madness could be produced in a sufficiently weak "recipient," especially if the "agent" keeps up his or her "enchantments" for a prolonged period from the "deepest mind." The Viennese dream investigator, Dr. Wilhelm STEKEL, reached the conclusion on the basis of his materials that we would run short of gallows if poets were to be punished for all the crimes they have dreamed.[115]

Christian MORGENSTERN (1871–1914) warns—in the same vein as HARTMANN—against over-addiction to "tail forces," as the esoteric Taoists call them: "How many avalanches in the high Alps are caused by the leaping chamois! Remember this when you are clambering on the mountains of thought—and congratulate or blame yourself for them, or do both at once, according to your nature!"[116]

CHEVREUIL'S PENDULUM EXPERIMENTS

The New Thought axiom of William Walter ATKINSON (1862–1932) "Thoughts are things" finds its easiest proof in Chevreuil's Pendulum Experiments.[117] I shall repeat something I said about them in my Parapsychological Researches, etc.:[36] "They are named for the French chemist Michel Eugène CHEVREUIL (1786–1889), however the same experiment was performed earlier by the English explorer and scientist Sir Francis GALTON (1822–1911).

A large circle is described on paper and various radii are drawn inside it (a *trochos,* Greek for "wheel"). Then a ring, tied to a silk thread held between the thumb and finger of the right hand, is suspended motionless over the center of the circle. One

---

[115]KANKELEIT, p. 41; STEKEL, Dr. Wilhelm, *Der telepathische Traum* [The Telepathic Dream], *Die okkulte Welt collection,* No. 2 (Pfullingen, ca. 1920).

[116]MORGENSTERN, Christian, *Stufen* [Stages] (Munich, 1928).

[117]CHEVREUIL, Michel Eugène, *De la baguette divinatoire, du pendule dit explorateur et des tables tournantes* [The Divining Rod, the So-Called Exploratory Pendulum and Table Turning] (Paris, 1854).

[36]See earlier footnote, page 14.

thinks: let the pendulum swing to and fro in this or that direction, and the "rotating divining rod" (as Julie Böss Kniese called it) obeys. The direction [the "wheel-spoke" or radius over which the pendulum swings] can be altered at will by a change of thought (in other words, "ideomotorically").

"The old name 'wishing rod' still makes sense to us, not because we can grant wishes with it, but because in the hands of a believer . . . it responds to the slightest wish."[118] The "ideomuscular" motion of the pendulum can be turned to account in psychotherapy.[119] What is more, one can work up to the standard exercise of *inducing heaviness* in "Autogenic Training" [devised by Dr. Johannes Schultz (1884–1970). *Tr.*] with this phenomenon (Ousby).

When left to itself and temporarily released from the body as an operational unit, the right arm (the left arm in left-handers) can function as a pendulum. Lie down, raise the arm and desire a certain direction of swing. The consumption of nervous energy is much greater in working with the "arm pendulum" than it is with the sidereal pendulum.[120]

Indeed, the whole body can serve as a pendulum. A "swaying exercise" of the Schlaffhorst-Andersen School of Singing and Voice-production in the Heide bei Celle, was performed by standing with the feet firmly planted on the floor while describing circles with the body, arms stretched to their fullest extent, while imagining that one is a blade of grass swaying in the wind, or a rippling cornfield.[121]

Engineer Johannes Zacharias[122] and school principal Dr. Welisch (Graz) extended the simple Chevreuil pendulum test:

He invited a pendulist who was unknown to him to leave the audience and join him on the stage, placed himself behind

---

[118]Scheminzky, Ferdinand, "Wünschelrutenkunde" [Divining-Rod Science], *Lehrmeister-Bücherei*, No. 589–590), p. 34, Leipzig n.d.

[119]Graeter, Dr. Karl, *Menschenleiden als Lebensgeheimnis* [Human Suffering as Life's Secret] (Kandern (Bad.), 1926), p. 80, 170 f.

[120]Hemar, Otto, "Der Mensch als Pendel" [The Human Being as a Pendulum], *Astrale Warte* (1932), October issue.

[121]Kükelhaus, Hans, *Urzahl und Gebärde* [Basic Counting and Gesture] (Berlin, 1934), p. 240.

[122]Zacharias, J., *Rätsel der Natur* [The Riddle of Nature] (Munich, 1920), p. 30.

this person at a remove of about 5 or 6 paces, held in his hand a diagram on which 8 different oscillation paths were indicated, and got a control person to touch one of these lines silently with a finger. Without saying a word or making any kind of movement—but only by an act of will, WELISCH caused the deliberately passive pendulist, or his pendulum as the case may be, to swing in the direction chosen by the control person. This is a highly significant experiment in a positive or negative sense for the whole of research into the pendulum and the divining rod. It demonstrates the possibility of influencing the rod and pendulum telepathically."[123]

Furthermore, doubt is cast on the reliability of the sidereal pendulum as a "radiation indicator" since there are only a very few individuals who can (almost) completely empty their minds, especially for any length of time. It also becomes clear why even capable and competent dowsers are sure to fail in front of prejudiced and hostile committees.[124]

An experiment basically similar to that of ZACHARIAS and WELISCH was described more than a hundred years ago by the animal magnetist LAFONTAINE as an *anneau magique* (magic ring): "Shortly before the test the operator odically impregnates a gold ring with his hand, and then asks another person to hold the ring suspended by a silk thread over a tumbler half-full of water. Finally he places himself behind his subject, and by directing his fluid—with intention—makes the ring strike the side of the glass he visualized but did not mention to his subject."[125] The ring suspended on a thread as a divinatory device is as old as the divining rod (Latin: *virgula divina*; French: *baguette divinatoire*; German: *Wünschelrute*). Judah, one of the twelve sons of Jacob, left his ring, his cord, and his staff ("Moses rod"; forked branch) as a pledge for payment for an hour of love.[126]

---

[123]SURYA, G. W., *Okkulte Diagnostik und Prognostik* [Occult Diagnosis and Prognosis] (Lorch i. W., 1950), p. 131.

[124]RINGGER, p. 33 f.; GADICKE, Ing. Wilh., *Das siderische Pendel, die Wünschelrute und andere sid. Detektoren etc.* [The Sidereal Pendulum, the Divining Rod, and Other Sidereal Detectors, etc.] (Bad Oldesloe, 1924), p. 67.

[125]LAFONTAINE, p. 322 f.

[126]GENESIS, 38.

As a simple "mantic" (erroneously: "magic") device, the Galton-Chevreuil pendulum is called "sidereal" nowadays. It represents a "sensor of nerve-excitation" according to the Swiss geologist Prof. Albert HEIM (1849–1937), and "a stand-pipe rising out of the subconscious" according to Dr. Rudolf TISCHNER (born 1879).

ODIC JAMMERS

The oscillation of the pendulum can be inhibited merely by the presence of an odically strong individual—without the need for any telepathic action on the part of the latter. Thus the Zürich electrical engineer, E. K. MÜLLER observed "without a shadow of doubt" in 1912 that the "big strapping wife" of Privy Counsellor E. von PYCHLAU, M. D. (St. Petersburg) *had only to come up close to her husband* to cause the pendulum in his hand to stop. "The lady withdrew, and almost immediately his pendulum started working again."[127]

TELEPATHIC JAMMERS

There are also involuntary "telepathic jammers." Thus, the mere presence of my daughter, who is so like me, disturbs owing to her "strong-mindedness" any work on which I am concentrating, whereas the presence of my wife, who is my polar complement and lives more in her emotions, does not bother me. It is also a well-known fact that most people cannot bear it when someone stands behind them while they are working.[124]

This is so even when the worker is self-confident and the spectator is neither a critic nor someone with different ideas, but is simply watching without comment.

---

[127]MÜLLER, E. K., p. 4.
[124]See earier note, page 42.

Telepathic Therapy

I shall take as typical the procedure of Horatio W. Dresser (Boston), because, for one thing, he is not partisan, "no practitioner of spiritual healing," as he himself says; and for another thing, he is "only a searcher for truth" who publishes "the results of fifteen years' observations, during which he has had the privilege of seeing the successful employment of the principles he recommends." The numbers in square brackets are those of the booklets published in German in 1902.[128] Dresser takes as his starting point: "In every case of pain and disease we may assume that some sort of tension is present, an apprehensive uneasy gazing into the future, and impetuous urgent wishes . . . we are everlastingly wishing . . . that someone would come or that something would happen, and this *continual dissatisfaction results in an equally continual dissipation of energy*" [18].

And with the above sentence the remedy is also revealed: "If this tension can be removed, the resistance to the forces of nature will cease, too" [18–19]. Dresser suspects that there are such things as "psychosomatic" diseases: "Even conceding that a given complaint is a physical illness, if we wish to describe it as such, the fact remains that all this is conveyed to us entirely through the conscious mind . . . our conscious mind is equally responsible to repair what it has done, so that a new and healthier direction is taken" [20]. But if the patient can no longer perform this *metanoia* (Greek for "change of mind"), then the spiritual healer must initiate it on his or her behalf.

Dresser knows the value of friendly encouragement—"But we shall assume that the average patient, of whom we speak, *requires the help of a good listener as much as anything* [10–11]. The patient comes with the compliant attitude already described. The healer is in a 'sympathetic' frame of mind. . . . He asks no questions and does not allow any rehearsal of symptoms or aches

---

[128]Dresser, Horatio W., *Methoden und Probleme der geistigen Heilbehandlung* [The Methods and Problems of Spiritual Healing] (Leipzig, 1902).

and pains, which would serve only to freshen the misgivings, fears, and the mental picture. What is past is past, and the patient must simply concentrate on an ideal future. The healer sits near the patient and requests the latter to be quiet and receptive. The patient must try to achieve this state, not by hard effort, but as restfully as possible, and preferably should be concentrating on the practitioner rather than on himself or herself. The healer now turns his mind away from the noisy outside world and, as far as possible, shuts out sound, light, and physical sensations, and rises into the kingdom of the inner self or soul" [12]. This requires practice.

"However, often one and the same formula, as for example: 'In Him we live and move and have our being,' is found to be the most helpful thought as we immerse ourselves in silence. And often the same words or suggestions will be used to gain control over your own minds and to calm the agitated *atmosphere* of the patient, namely 'Still, still, be still!'"

"Nevertheless, in spiritual healing, there is certainly no attempt to transmit certain thoughts, nor any effort to master or hypnotize the patient's mind. Rather a soft, tranquilizing atmosphere should emanate from the healer so that the patient can absorb from it whatever is needed or is capable of being received." (The biologist and philosopher, Professor Hans DRIESCH (1867–1941) used to speak of "entering into possession of the contents of another consciousness.") The healer is not the almighty factor but only the instrument of the Higher Power. "His endeavor is to become open and free in spirit and then to produce the same condition in the patient" [13].

"Even if at the start of treatment one knows nothing about what the patient is suffering, the seat of the trouble will soon become apparent to the healer, because the thought aimed at the patient will run into this blockage" [15]. The spiritual healer "focuses his force" on it. "One must not permit oneself to be obstructed by symptoms and doubts, but must look to the ultimate goal and to that of the patient as he or she should be—in good health, balanced, restful, and strong. *One must hold the right thoughts more firmly in mind than the patient holds wrong thoughts*" [15–16].

I figure that the spiritual healer would be encouraged to think "right thoughts" by the following quotation from J. Ellis BARKER (born 1870): "Health is natural, sickness is not. Therefore the potential for health is inside us." In reply to the question: "But how can this realization of the divine ideal, union with God through spiritual concentration, extend itself to another individual and bring about the same expansion?" DRESSER [p. 21] uses the following illustration: "The best explanation of the process is the transmission of musical vibrations. When two pianos occupy adjacent rooms and a note is sounded on one of them, the string in the other that is tuned to the same pitch will be set vibrating." From this example we can see quite clearly that as long ago as 1902 DRESSER had the concept of "resonance"! In 1922, Dr. Paul VAGELER declared: "Suggestion is resonance in the receptive brains of others,"[69] and in 1951 Dr. Josef GEMASSMER spoke of "meditational resonance,"[129] though neither had heard of the Bostonian. Having now, I imagine, shown something about the reality of "animal magnetism" and telepathy, I can examine the question of whether we are dealing with biological emanations or with thought waves.

PURE ODIC PHENOMENA

A pure, that is to say, an *unmixed*, odic phenomenon is present (first and foremost involving people but also in a quite general sense) when there is "**health by contagion**" as TENZEL (1629), BUTTENSTEDT[130] (ca. 1895), and JAEGER (1908) term it; when the grandmother who sleeps with her grandchild becomes fat and flourishing while the little one grows thin and weak;[131] when the "seeress of Prevorst" (Kr. Gronau i. Württ.), Christina

---

[69]See earlier footnote, page 25.
[129]ROWE, Harvey T., "Du wirst gesund durch Ekstase!" [Regain Your Health in Trance!] *Neue Post* (1951), 21 [May 26], 1 f.
[130]BUTTENSTEDT, Carl, *Die Übertragung der Nervenkraft: Ansteckung durch Gesundheit* [The Transmission of Nerve Force: Infection by Health] (Rüdersdorf bei Berlin, ca. 1895).
[131]HAUPT, Dr. Hermann, *Die strahlende Lebenskraft und ihre Gesetze* [The radiating vital force and its laws] (Althofnaß bei Breslau, 1922), p. 43.

Friederica HAUFFE (1801–1829) née WANNER,[132] Kaspar HAUSER the mysterious foundling,[17] and spiritualistic mediums attract forces ("Od vampires") from their environment that even make them ill; when DU PREL tells of a dying woman who revived as soon as her husband (who had previously mesmerized her) entered the room and always fell back lifelessly as soon as he left it;[133] when in 1949 the then chief of police in Munich, Franz Xavier PITZER stated that his chronic sciatica had undergone a radical improvement in the presence of the healer Bruno GRÖNING (Grönkowsky, 1906–1959);[134] when in 1949 the Marburg professor of psychology, Dr. FISCHER, sat in GRÖNING'S chair in the HÜLSMANN home in Herford and, at the very moment he sat down, felt a severe pain in the region of his right kidney, together with palpitations of the heart and shortage of breath"— earlier his right kidney had been repeatedly inflamed.[135]

Also consider sympathetic symptoms—**Infection with disease (morbid substances)**. We have "odic infection with disease" when Professor Johann VELDEN-PLAN describes cases of secondary nicotine poisoning of husband or wife sharing the same bed and also of the children.[136] [This could be due to what we now call "passive smoking." Tr.]

When Dr. CALLEDO in Noputo, lacking an antidote, resuscitated someone poisoned by opium after two hours of continuous "magnetizing," he himself fell into a coma lasting many hours, and even three days later, in spite of frequent cups of strong coffee, he still exhaled the odor of laudanum.[137]

Mummial infection involving animals: one can gain the friendship of animals (e.g., dogs and even tigers!) by giving them bread to eat that has been held under one's armpit to soak up the

---

[132]KERNER, Justinus, *Die Seherin von Prevorst* [The Seeress of Prevorst] (Stuttgart, 1829, Reclam, No. 3315–3320).

[17]See earlier footnote, page 5.

[133]DU PREL, Baron Dr. Carl, "Die Magie als Naturwissenschaft" [Magic as Science], *Arch. thier. Magn. I*: 140, II, p. 29. (Leipzig, 1920).

[134]DE VAIRE, Gaston, "Bruno Gröning, der berühmte Heilspender" [Bruno Gröning, the Celebrated Healer], p. 32 [after a report by Dr. Kurt TRAMPLER, *Münchener Allgemeine*, September 7, 1949].

[135]VAIRE, pp. 29–30.

[136]Private communication.

[137]BUTTENSTEDT, p. 128.

sweat, and by frequently spitting saliva into their mouths, as all the Renaissance "Books of Knowledge" agree.[138] The vehicle for Od (here the sweat-soaked bread) was at that time known as "mummy." Thus one could speak of "mummial infection." Dog breeders assure me that it works.

When the butcher's lady assistants are bursting with health and the butcher's men never become consumptive, this can be attributed to the odic emanation from the red meat and says something about the obsolete "animal baths"—*balnea animalia*[139]—which were once recommended by even the greatest physicians.[140] Something on the same lines is the attempt to enrich the body fluids by inhaling the gasified blood of a male lamb.[141]

Mummification of dead meat occurs as well. For example, in 1913 Dr. Gaston DURVILLE (Paris) mummified a corpse's hand by magnetic treatment,[142] Mme. X. in 1912 produced odorless desiccated oysters by irradiating them or touching them with her hands,[143] in 1928 the "pictographer" Heinrich NÜSSLEIN (1879–1947) exhibited at the Kornburg bei Nuremberg dozens of pieces of meat, fishes, and birds, that he had petrified over the years by the radiation from his hands,[144] and the archivist and

---

[138]TENZEL, Andreas, *Medicina diastatica oder in die Ferne würkende Arzney-Kunst* [Medicina Diastatica, or the Medical Art Practiced from a Distance] (Leipzig u. Hof, 1629, 1753), pp. 140, 141; GLOREZ, Andreas, *Eröffnetes Wunderbuch usw.* [The Unsealed Book of Wonders, etc.] (Regensburg u. Stadtamhof, 1700), p. 78.

[139]DE VÈZE Bosc, *Traité de la Longévité* [A Treatise on Longevity] (Paris, 1908), pp. 28–29; CARUS, pp. 83, 115.

[140]CARUS, pp. 83, 115; HUFELAND, Christoph Wilhelm, *Makrobiotik oder die Kunst, das menschliche Leben verlängern* [Macrobiotics or the Art of Prolonging Human Life], 1796.

[141]SCHRÖDTER, Willy, *Magie/Geister/Mystik* [Magic/Spirits/Mysticism] (Berlin, 1958), pp. 113, 178.

[142]HARTMANN, A., "Haltbarmachung und Mumienbildung einer menschlichen Hand" ["The Preservation and Mummification of a Human Hand], *Z. Heilmagnetismus* (1930), 8 [August issue].

[143]GROBE-WUTISCHKY, Arthur, *Fakirwunder und moderne Wissenschaft* [Fakir Wonders and Modern Science] (Berlin-Pankow, 1923), p. 66; FREUDENBERG, Dr. F., "Über ungewöhnliche aus dem Körper ausstrahlende Kräfte" [Strange Forces Propagated by the Body] (*Z. Revalo-Bund*, 1925, April issue); Anonymous, "Die Madame-X-Strahlen" [The Madam-X-rays], *Zbl. Okk.* (1913), May issue: 612.

[144]FEKL, Franz Karl, "Heinrich Nüßlein, der okkulte Maler von Nürnberg" [Heinrich Nüßlein, the Occult Painter of Nuremberg], *Zbl. Okk.* (1928), February issue: 372.

mesmerist Dr. Karl BERTRAM (born 1878) successfully ran the same tests in Berlin-Steglitz during and after 1931.[145]

As regards **mummification of plants**: the two last-named individuals petrified flowers and vegetables (*loc. cit.*). And even today there are certain gardeners who have a specially "lucky" hand—a **green thumb**. As regards the brief time in which the seeds are held in their "golden hands" as they call them in China,[146] or "sunshine hands" as they say in Germany, compare the time of exposure to HILDEBRAND'S and HEERMANN'S "growth rays"!

Blood offerings to the Dryads—when potted plants in butchers' shops grow amazingly well.[139] [". . . and in the midst of the tree sat a friendly old woman with a very peculiar dress; it was green, like the elder leaves, and figured all over with elder-flowers, so that at first sight it was difficult to make out whether it was really stuff, or the living green and flowers of the tree. 'What is the woman's name?' the little boy asked. 'Well the Romans and Greeks called her Dryad, but that is a name we do not understand,' the old man said, 'We have a better name for her. We call her Mother-elder.'" "Mother-Elder," *Andersen's Fairy Tales*: English trans., S. W. Partridge, London, ca. 1913. *Tr. note*].

PURE TELEPATHIC PHENOMENA

A pure, that is to say, an *unmixed* telepathic phenomenon is present, when according to WILLIAM OF PARIS (1210–1273) someone senses in advance the homecoming of a loved one from two miles away;[147] when ladies belonging to the heretical *Alumbrados*

---

[145]BERTRAM, Dr. Karl, "Der Mensch als Sender" [Humans as Transmitters], *Pranabuch*, No. 21 (Pfullingen I. W.: n.d., ca. 1920), pp. 56–58; Anonymous, "Der Mensch als Sender," *Wiss. u. Fschr.* (1933), April issue), 39 f.

[146]FRICHET, Henri, *La Médecine et l'Occultisme en Chine* [Medicine and Occultism in China] (Paris n.d.), p. 110.

[139]See earlier footnote, page 48.

[147]AGRIPPA, vol. I, p. 260; SCHRÖDTER, *Offenbarungen* [Revelations], p. 28.

in Spain perceived a passing priest from their rooms without see-ing him;[148] when in the winter of 1862–1863 Helene VON DÖNNIGES (1845–1911) sensed the presence of her beloved, Ferdinand LAS-SALLE (1825–1864) in a crowded ballroom by a sudden surge of "a sort of joyful apprehension";[149] when Marie CORELLI (1864–1924), who most probably was unaware of the above-mentioned fact, depicted in 1886 in her sensational first novel the same incident in regard to her character, the Italian painter Raffaelo CELLINI.[150] ["I was standing near the large open window of the ballroom, conversing with one of my recent partners, when a sudden inex-plicable thrill shot through me from head to foot. Instinctively I turned, and saw Cellini approaching."]

Again, telepathic phenomena occur when, in 1876, Dr. NEW-TON (according to SURYA: Stephenson) of San Francisco elicited an unexpected curative "electric shock" from Dr. Franz HARTMANN who was then staying in Texas;[151] when in 1884 Mark TWAIN found that he knew the contents of an unopened letter that had come in response to his own intense thoughts—a fact submitted by him to the Society for Psychical Research in London;[152] when at about the same time Joseph Alexandre Marquis SAINT-YVES D'ALVEYDRE (1842–1909) was in permanent astral contact ("com-munion") with his wife, so that his heart stopped for a moment when she fainted a long way away, and conversely she felt it when he pricked himself with a needle.[153]

A fairly recent example of fused feelings (Greek: *neurogamos* = nerve marriage) is that of English landscape painter Arthur SEVERN, whose upper lip was injured at seven o'clock in the morning when he was on board his yacht and there was a sud-den shift of wind. His wife, who had stayed at home, awoke feeling that she had received a heavy blow on the mouth and

[148]LLORCA, Bernardino, S. J., *Die spanische Inquisition und die Alumbrados* [The Spanish In-quisition and the Alumbrados] (Berlin and Bonn, 1934), p. 55.
[149]VON RACOWITZA, Helene (Dönniges), *Von Anderen und mir: Erinnerungen aller Art* [Others and Myself: Memories of All Kinds] (Berlin 1909/10, 1918); NIELSEN, p. 181.
[150]CORELLI, *A Romance of Two Worlds* (New York, n.d.), p. 48.
[151]HARTMANN, *Denkwürdige Erinnerungen* [Remarkable Memories], pp. 146–148.
[152]NIELSEN, p. 243 f.
[153]STRINDBERG, August, *Ein neues Blaubuch* [A Second Blue Book] (Munich, 1920), p. 807.
[154]TENHAEFF, W. H. C., *Außergewöhnliche Heilkräfte* [Unusual Healing Powers] (Olten u. Freiburg I. Br., 1957), p. 118 f.

found herself bleeding from her upper lip![154] Cornelius Agrippa would not have found such cases particularly surprising, for he says: "The emotional bond between many lovers is so strong that what one suffers is also endured by the other."[155]

In identical twins, neurogamy is especially frequent and far-reaching (in both senses of the word), for there is a close telepathic tie between them. A pertinent example was reported in *Bild* on November 25, 1958:

BOY SHARES HIS BROTHER'S PAIN

Tomorrow, when in the English port of Newcastle upon Tyne little Keith Main *(aged 5) comes under the surgeon's knife for a hole in the heart operation, his twin brother* Kenneth *will be kept under close observation by the doctors—the reason being that one twin always feels any pain inflicted on the other. In the hospital last week, as a preliminary operation was being performed on Keith, Kenneth suddenly cried out loud at home and fell almost unconscious into the arms of his mother. The hands of the clock pointed to 11:32. This was the exact second when the operation on his twin brother began in the nearby hospital. And yet Keith knew nothing of his brother's operation.*

Our scientific correspondent comments:
Where uniovular (identical) twins are concerned, even scientists occasionally talk of a linked destiny. And often it appears that in some mysterious way the thoughts and fortunes of one twin are conveyed to the other.

The above statement made by the scientific correspondent on the shared fate of twins, only helps to bear out that "identical twins are in especially close telepathic communication."

INDUCTION THROUGH EMPATHY

Another example: in 1888, during an evening lecture delivered in Watkins, NY, HARTMANN was unintentionally freed from a

---

[155]AGRIPPA, vol. I, p. 305.

toothache that had been caused by a chill. The young spiritual healer, J. W., was unknown to him. He participated in the mental life of the young lady as long as her influence lasted;[156] this was *âveçah* (Sanskrit: soul-grafting; Hebrew: 'ibbur[157]), and the German doctor experienced the charm of the participation mystique of Lucien LÉVY-BRUHL (1857–1939).

SPIRITUAL HEALING IN THE USA

In 1902, DRESSER urged the spiritual healer to adopt a "sympathetic frame of mind"—or, as Ralph Waldo TRINE (1866–1958) would have said, to be "in tune with the infinite"[158] and then to induce this state in the patient by "resonance."[159]

"HE CLOTHED HIMSELF WITH CURSING LIKE AS WITH HIS GARMENT" (PS. 109: 18)

In 1922, Eira HELLBERG (born in 1884) gave an eyewitness account of how the *stream of hatred* projected by an envious masseuse almost killed a female patient in a sanatorium in Baden-Baden, even after the primary cause of the illness had been removed. The sufferer could sense the exact moment when her "ill-wisher" entered or left the building.[160] In 1944, lively Maria HAIDER sud-

---

[156]HARTMANN, *Denkwürdige Erinnerungen* [Remarkable Memories], p. 49 f.

[157]OPPERMANN, A. M., *Die Yoga-Aphorismen des Patanjali* (Leipzig, 1925), Verse 38, p. 73. ["When the cause of bondage is removed, the yogi can, by knowledge of the nervous system, concentrate his mind upon the body of another and enter into it." *Aphorisms of Yoga*, translated by Shree Purohit Swami with an introduction by W. B. Yeats (London: Faber & Faber, 1938, new edition 1973), p. 70; MEYRINK, Gust., *Walpurgisnacht* [ch. "Aweysha"] (Bremen, 1917), pp. 133–158; SCHRÖDTER, Willy, *Offenbarungen* [Revelations], pp. 29–30; and "Einfühlung" [Empathy], *Neue Wiss.* (1957), 2 [Aug./Sept./Oct.], 82 f.; MRSICH, Dr. Wilhelm, "Die Erweckung des übersinnlichen Wahrnehmungsvermögens" [The Awakening of the Supersensual Faculties of Perception] *Mensch. u. Schicksal* (1957), 5 [May]: 7–14.

[158]DRESSER, p. 7.

[159]DRESSER, p. 13.

[160]HELLBERG, p. 90 f.

denly fainted while walking in the park in Mährisch-Ostrau, and later learned that on the same day (August 12) and at the same hour, her elder brother had been shot in the chest and fatally wounded.[161]

MAGNETIZING ALWAYS HAS TELEPATHIC COMPONENTS

Where impressions *having a certain intent* are made by someone supercharged with Od—the *sahala* of the Toba-Batak in Sumatra[162]—a telepathic component is invariably present and deserves notice. A knowledge of this inevitable double flow appears in the words of Cornelius AGRIPPA (1510): "The body and mind of one person can be worked on by the anima of a second person because the mind is far more powerful, strong, fervent, and brisk than the vapors that flow from the body."[163]

When, from 1964 onward, Dr. Paul VASSE (Amiens/Somme) and his wife have "forced" the germination and growth of plant seeds by concentrated thought, and when Dr. Richard DE SILVA of the Medical Research Institute in Ceylon (now Sri Lanka) reported on November 9, 1953, at the Sixth International Congress for Microbiology in Rome, the successful inhibition by concentrated thought of the growth of bacterial cultures, as I have already described in detail elsewhere, we are inclined to imagine that thought projection was primary in both cases. However, Roger BACON (1214–1294) said: *Natura enim obedit cogitationibus et vehementibus desideriis animae.*[164] [It is a fact that nature obeys the thoughts and ardent desires of the soul]. In the second case (that of inhibited bacterial growth), the concentrated thoughts negatively infected the odic emanations from the eyes—which were

---

[161]Heading, "Das Kaleidoskop. Menschen/Schicksale/Mysterien" [The Kaleidoscope. People/Fates/Mysteries] in *Neue Ill. Wochenschau* (1958), 27 [August 8].
[162]WINKLER, Dr. Johs., *Die Toba-Batak auf Sumatra in gesunden und kranken Tagen* [The Toba-Batak in Sumatra on Healthy and Unhealthy Days] (Stuttgart, 1925), p. 3.
[163]AGRIPPA, vol. I, p. 316.
[164]BACON, Roger, *De mirabili potestate artis et naturae* [Concerning the Marvelous Powers of Art and Nature].

fixed on the object for a long time. The "ocular rays," which since 1921 have even been said to be measurable,[165] were secondary, but worked in tandem with the thought-waves.

Cures brought about by the silent presence of the healer (and these are still happening) must therefore be termed *sit venia verbo* [if I may be allowed the expression]—"combined actions."

GEMASSMER'S NATURAL FORCE METHOD

In my opinion, this is shown exceptionally clearly by Dr. GEMASS-MER'S "power of nature method," of which he himself said in 1951: "The core of it is this, that I place myself in a state of inner consciousness that enables me to take into myself the 'great power of nature,' which I then transmit to the patient."[166] The Tyrolean yogi-doctor has given the illuminating name "meditational ecstasy" to this "core" of self-absorption. What is implied by this is that it is not some unemotional, sterile act of thought, but emotional forces that are mobilized by meditation and enable us to "tune in to the wavelengths being broadcast by the universe." The "great power of nature," which flows into the receptacle that has been opened for it, is then conveyed to the (odically deficient) sufferer by the laying on of hands, or by magnetic passes, as the case may be. This procedure is called "meditative resonance," an epithet signifying receptivity in the patient.

GEMASSMER also defines the "great power of nature" as "life currents."[167] To me, it is the macrocosmic, non-specific, universal Od, which becomes transformed into human Od when passing through the microcosmic man or woman. Paul SÉDIR (Yvon Leloup,

---

[165]"Augenstrahlen werden gemessen" [Occular Rays Have Been Measured], *Zbl. Okk.* (1932), December issue, 232, 249 f.; Russ, Charles, "An Instrument that is Set in Motion by Vision or the Proximity of the Human Body," in *The Lancet*, (30.7.1921), p. 222; (6.8.1921), p. 308; (13.8.1921), p. 361 f.; KELLER, Dr. A., *Magnetismus—die Urheilkraft des Menschen* [Magnetism—The Primary Human Healing Power] (Cademario, 1959), p. 24. [See also, WILSON, Colin, *Strange Powers* (London: Latimer New Dimensions Limited, 1973), pp. 27–28.
[166]ROWE, p. 1.
[167]GEMASSMER, Dr. Joseph, "Die geistigen Heilweisen im Gutachten eines Arztes" [A Doctor's Verdict on Spiritual Healing], *Die weiße Fahne* (1953), 1 [January], 47–48.

1871–1926) speaks of the *Lumière astrale humanisée* [the humanized astral light],[168] which puts the phenomenon in a nutshell, because from the days of Franz Anton MESMER (1733–1815) until now, the practitioners of healing magnetism "humanize" the electric currents of healing magnetism by connecting themselves to them, and they then pass them on to their patients by the laying on of hands.[169] GEMASSMER switches on the "life currents" by entering into a state of ecstasy through meditation. Meanwhile, the person seeking a cure lies physically relaxed and inwardly expectant. In themselves, the objects of meditation (the pictorial imagery) used by the meditator will not fail to create a resonance in percipients who have placed themselves in a receptive frame of mind—even if the response is only a vague feeling. Many individuals, however, even catch sight internally of the meditator's pictorial imagery.

This seems to have been exemplified in the case (studied by the Munich parapsychologist Prof. Karl GRUBER (1881–1927), of the factory manager's wife, M.T., whose children repeatedly picked up, without knowing it, as they lay dreaming, the thoughts, feelings, and mental imagery that came into their mother's mind when she was reading in the evenings.[170] As excitation is gradually intensified by hidden agents—and inspirational enthusiasm is a form of excitation—emotional transference in the patients will probably become increasingly marked. Indians speak of the prayer "to evoke Brahma." The only way in which anyone can be evoked is by an evocation acting on one who is capable of being evoked (a process of induction!).

If we use the word "prayer" in a broad sense, as Lord Edward George BULWER-LYTTON (1803–1873) does in his favorite work *Zanoni* (1842), meditation may be equated with prayer. In "Book the Seventh, chapter the seventeenth and last" he writes: "The thoughts of souls that would aspire as mine, are *all prayer.*"

---

[168]SÉDIR, Paul, *Histoire et Doctrines des Rose-Croix* (Bihorel-lez-Rouen (p. 1), 1932), p. 210.

[169]KLUGE, §125, p. 146; DE ROCHAS, Alb., *Die Ausscheidung des Empfindungsvermögens* [The Transference of the Power of Perception] (Leipzig, 1909), p. 381. DU PREL, vol. II, p. 36; VÖCKLER, R. and SPAHRMANN, F., "Erwiederung auf die Prof. Eckhoff, Ob.-Ing. Meiersche Flugschrift" [A Reply to the Pamphlet of Prof. Eckhoff and Chief-Engineer Meier], *Zarch. Pendelforsch.* (1933) 1–2: 10.

[170]Anonymous, "Vererbung durch Telepathie" [Telepathic Transmission] *Der Mittag* (1926), 280 [December 1].

I can well imagine that—as Prof. Wilhelm H. C. TENHAEFF (born 1894) says, "in many cases it turns out (when we look into it) that during the treatment session practitioner and patient form a peculiar bipartite unit, a *bipersonnalité*,[171] a *sympsychismus*, or a *diapsychicum*.

POSITIVE MENTAL PICTURES

The mental imagery used by the therapist to help relax and inspire himself or herself has to be personally appealing. GEMASS-MER suggests that it should be scenery of some kind.[167] At all events, experienced psychagogues advise us to relax with mental pictures of a waving cornfield or a billowing sea, "which in spite of their apparent restlessness are restful to look at."[172]

In my considered opinion, internal imagery can be replaced by external, blank-minded absorption in the continually shape-shifting ocean of clouds.[173] Or by gazing at some external picture that has made a deep impression on one, such as the wonderful face of the Madonna, which is so chaste and harmonious.[172] Or by dwelling on an affecting, pregnant quotation (Indian: *japam*), such as the following, which is a great favorite of mine, although I no longer remember who wrote it: "A little hamlet full of forgotten voices. There one hears the clock striking at noon . . . as if from some far-off time."

Another example is the stillness-exhaling sentence of Adalbert STIFTER (1805–1868), which is so reminiscent of a Japanese *haiku*: "A tom-cat walked along the house-ridge and looked up at

---

[171]TENHAEFF, p. 277; BUTTERSACK, Dr. Felix, *Körperloses Leben: Diapsychicum* [Incorporeal Life: Diapsychicum]. (Leipzig, 1936).

[167]See earlier footnote, page 54.

[172]RADO, Kurt (Niels Kampmann), *Seelische Hemmungen* [Mental Inhibitions] (Kampen/Sylt, 1922), p. 39; LEHMANN, Gustav, *Wie ich meine Nervosität verlor* [How I Overcame My Nervousness] (Natural self-help for nervousness through self-suggestion in the waking state according to the method of Dr. Paul Emile LÉVY of Nancy) (Leipzig, 1909), p. 23.

[173]SCHRÖDTER, Willy, "Wolken" [Clouds], *Natur und Kultur* (1957), IV: 213 f.; and "Kultur der Stille" [The Cultivation of Tranquillity], *Neues Licht* (1952), vol. III: 58–59).

[172]See earlier footnote, above.

the moon; a faint silvery haze drifted over the roofs of the distant town; it seemed to be growing quieter every minute."

I think that the operator can "tune" himself or herself musically, too (II Kings 3: 15), and can induce a "nirvana-like" frame of mind by the "Autogenic training"[174] of neurologist Prof. Johannes SCHULTZ (born in Berlin-Charlottenburg in 1884), and could then transfer this frame of mind by induction to the recipients on synchronizing with them.

---

[174]SCHULTZ, Prof. J.H., *Das autogene Training* [Autogenic Training] (Leipzig, 1934); and *Übungsheft für das autogene Training* [Autogenic Training Workbook] (Leipzig, 1935).

PSYCHOSOMATIC DISEASES

The primary indications for curative emotional transfers are the psychosomatic diseases. "It was not the fact of a cure that impressed us, but the unmistakable evidence that the psychic or spiritual change preceded the somatic. . . . The potentialities of Subud in helping psychopathic conditions are still almost wholly unexplained" BENNETT.[175]

The typical indications for such a curative emotional transfer or "regenerative impulse" will, to begin with, probably have to be sought among the host of psychosomatic diseases.[176] and I always assume that the telepath does not stay *tele* (Greek, far) from the patient, but remains in his or her immediate presence. Since there is no manual contact in this form of treatment it may still be classed as remote healing. Literal "treatment at a distance" assumes an emotional affinity that cannot be mass-produced and therefore, in general practice the cases where it occurs can be counted on the fingers of one hand. Dr. GEMASSMER said of it: "I use this only when a psychic contact exists that is so strong that the patient is present as an image inside me" (letter of July 26, 1953).

Only very exceptional healers who overflow with compassion and universal love can possibly make emotional contact with anyone at any distance. This must be seen as a grace arising out of saintly thoughts, speech, and actions, and it requires special legitimization. What is more, such Amtsleute Christi [Stewards of Christ] (PARACELSUS; I Corinthians 4: 1) do not need to "tune in" first, or to relax and elevate their thoughts, since they

[175]BENNETT, J.G., *Concerning Subud* (New York: University Books, 1959), pp. 69, 175; SCHRÖDTER, Willy, "Subud oder der Kontakt mit der Lebenskraft" [Subud or Contact with the Life-Force], *Neue Wiss.* (1959), 2 [March/April]: 67–74.
[176]ALKAN, L., "Anatomische Organerkrankungen aus seelischen Ursachen" [Anatomic organic diseases with psychological causes]. 1930.

maintain uninterrupted communion with the sacred—for their "conversation is in heaven" (Philippians 3: 20).

"I made a list for myself of those diseases it had been shown could (not must!) be psychosomatic, noting to which special affect in particular they could be traced. My various informants were in agreement in naming as such diseases: heart trouble, angina pectoris, high blood pressure, gastric and duodenal ulcers, biliousness, diabetes, exophthalmic goiter, gout, rheumatism, and asthma; and also a certain type of cold (*rhinitis vasomotoria*) and dental cavities due to a disturbance of the calcium balance in the body because of negative moods" (Dr. W.J.L. McGonigle).

One and the same psychological affect has actually been given for different diseases—which leads to the conclusion that it operates in each individual on a different *locus minoris resistentiae* [place of least resistance]. The prevailing opinion is that it is *always a negative affect*! Jealousy, revengeful thoughts, anger, grief, and fear in the most diverse forms, and a consequent refusal to face up to one's problems, are the main culprits.

Anxiety—Disease Multiplier No. 1

I personally am inclined, with Dresser,[128] Georges Barbarin[177] and Dr. I. Stewart, to see in fear and anxiety the "disease coefficient No. 1" or the "health-robber *par excellence*." According to press reports, the last-named, an English physician, has studied at the University Hospital in Bristol some 200 cases of high blood pressure. He was able to establish that, almost without exception, those patients who were aware of their condition lived in fear of apoplexy, and most of them complained of severe chronic headaches. However, those who did not know what was the matter with them had no headaches at all—or only occasional

---

[128]See earlier footnote, page 44.

[177]Barbarin, Georges, *La Peur—Maladie No. 1* [Anxiety—The No. 1 Disease] (Paris: Ed. de l'Ermite, 1949); Asturel, *Angst, unser Feind Nr. 1* [Anxiety, Our Enemy No. 1], new edition; Dr. C. M. Cobes (Talisman-Bücherei Bd. 1).

ones—even if their blood pressure was higher than that of the others! Stewart followed this up by making observations on inmates with other diseases, and obtained the enlightening result that persistent anxiety feelings should be regarded as the prime cause of recurrent headaches!

Psychosomatic diseases have always been recognized as such by the empirics. It is an interesting fact that from time immemorial empirics have always known about the potentially morbiferous influence of the psyche on the soma. Our common experience has been crystallized in the sentence, "It makes me sick!," said in reference to some unreasonable demand or hardship. To judge by what one hears in ordinary conversation, it is the stomach that suffers most in this regard. Thus someone will say: "I am sick to my stomach," or, "It has gone to my stomach," or, "It makes me nauseous," or even more bluntly, "I am fed up to the back teeth," or, "It makes me want to throw up." As far as the spleen and gall-bladder are concerned, we have the expressions: "He is venting his spleen," or, "She is jaundiced," or, "He is full of bile." One can suffer from nettle rash when one is ready to burst (out of one's skin) with rage over being ill-treated. Grief and sorrow are said to "squeeze the heart"—the same feeling as in *angina pectoris*! In Germany, fault-finding is blamed on an affection of the liver: "A louse must have crawled over his/her liver!"

Even science has occasionally described psychosomatic diseases with colloquial vividness, as in: "In exophthalmic goiter the thyroid gland weeps into the blood" (because of chronic hopelessness and lack of fulfillment); or, "Gastric ulcers result not from what we eat, but from what is eating us." The latter sentence so impressed James C. HAGERTY, the White House Press Secretary under President Dwight David EISENHOWER (born 1890), that he made a warning sign of it and stood it on his desk.

Experience teaches that, "consuming hatred can in certain circumstances produce a corrosive skin eruption (lupus)."[178] And excessive modesty has been known to produce barrenness, the so-called "protective sterility."

---

[178]SURYA, G. W. and STRAUSS, Dr. Alfred, *Theurgische Heilmethoden* [Theurgic Methods of Treatment] (Lorch I. W., 1936), pp. 75–86, footnote.

THE PSYCHIC COMPONENT STILL AWAITS DISCOVERY

It is entirely credible that *many* other diseases have psychic causes and that these causes will one day be revealed. Thus fifty years ago [i.e., ca. 1910. *Tr.*] the American doctor Sheldon LEAVITT, (1848–1933) maintained that, "Each disease starts as a psychosis."[179] And nearly a quarter of a century ago [i.e., in 1936. *Tr.*] Dr. Gerhard OCKEL (Guben) formulated his golden "Thoughts on organ-neuroses":

PHYSICAL ILLNESSES OF NEUROTIC ORIGIN ARE ERADICATED ONLY BY A RESTORATION OF THE PSYCHOLOGICAL BALANCE

When the psychological stress due to the vicissitudes of the patient's life is more than he or she can bear, a true organic neurosis is present (an organic dysfunction of neurotic origin). To anyone who has understood the inner connections, it is clear that the best that can be done by any palliative treatment of individual symptoms (such as fullness in the stomach, stabbing pains in the heart, giddiness, etc.) is only a temporary relief. To treat the stomach of a person with a gastric neurosis would be like treating a depressed or embittered person for "turned down mouth corners" and massaging the muscles of the mouth.[180] Every child knows that the corners of the mouth will automatically return to their normal position when the patient has shaken off depression or bitterness. A real and lasting cure of an organic neurosis is possible only when the source of the trouble (the disturbance of the psychic balance) is removed." [181]

The spiritual healer "must hold on to right thinking more tenaciously than the patient does to his or her wrong thinking."[182] "What the healer is trying to do is to become open and

---

[179]LEAVITT, Sheldon, *Wege zur Höhe* [Upward Paths] (Stuttgart, 1909), p. 239.

[180]KESSEMEIER, Heinrich, *Das andere Anlitz des Todes* [The Other Face of Death] (Hamburg, 1929), p.96 f.; "If the advocates of the physical causation theory were right, the lines of grief would etch themselves into the face before the spirit was downcast. But everyone knows that the reverse is true: and yet they refuse to draw the logical conclusion."

[181]OCKEL, Dr. Gerhard, "Gedanken über Organ-Neurosen" [Thoughts of Organic Neurosis], *Neuform-Rdsch*, 1936. 9 [September]: 228.

[182]DRESSER, pp. 15–16.

free in spirit and then to induce the same condition in the sufferer." Nevertheless, we should never lose sight of the fact that
"the healer is not the omnipotent factor, but only the willing
instrument of the Higher Power."[183] According to Eastern wisdom: "The Lord laughs on two occasions—when brothers divide
their land with a surveyor's chain and when the doctor says to
the patient, 'I will cure you!' " It was this realization that led the
Rosicrucian therapists to adopt as an axiom, "Not unto us, O
Lord, not unto us, but unto thy name give glory!" (Psalm 115, 1).

PHYSICAL AILMENTS HAVE PSYCHIC "MULTIPLIERS"

Without wishing to go as far as LEAVITT, we can agree with the
opinion of a certain Dr. Erwin LIEK (1878–1935) on the psychic
components or "accompanying chord" of every physical illness.
"The (physical) illness is also a psychic disease, and the healthy
psyche of the physician has to heal the sick psyche of the patient." Therefore "emotional transfer" should always be considered as a supplementary therapy. In *Subud Latihan*, BENNETT'S
experience was this:

> *It was not the fact of a cure that impressed us, but the unmis-
> takable evidence that the psychic spiritual change preceded
> the somatic. The healing of a distressed soul is more remark-
> able than recovery from an illness. When one sees the two in
> juxtaposition and can follow the course of the transition from
> the psychic to the somatic, one cannot doubt that a very great
> and a very good force is at work.*[175]

Thus, even in all those other diseases that one would not class as
psychosomatic, "emotional transfer" is useful as a *supplementary*
therapy if the relaxed and tranquil spirit of the healer is able to
infuse into the sufferer a peace so profound that mental interfer-

---

[183]DRESSER, p. 13.
[175]See earlier footnote, page 58.

ence with the recuperative power (or *vis medicatrix naturae* [the healing power of nature]) subsides and the latter is fully restored to the performance of its proper purposes.

So-Called "Distant Healing"

Not long after the first World War "distant" or "spiritual" healers began advertising their services in occult magazines. Their treatment consisted of this: at a certain hour in the evening the client was to adopt a receptive and passive frame of mind while the healer transmitted "currents of energy" to him or her. A picture, or even a specimen of the handwriting, of the patient served as a "contact point." Numerous testimonials certified cures of all possible diseases.

Far be it from me to dispute over, or cast doubt on, the success with which these "telepaths" are said to have "locked on" at the agreed time. However, I do maintain that (for reasons yet to be disclosed) even the best attempt to "lock on" could reach the proposed "receiver" in only a few cases, quite apart from the fact that precisely here "feeling is all" (Goethe), and feeling is not made to order.

It is another story with those spiritually advanced human beings (yet to be described) who can reach anybody at any time with their universal benevolence. In this connection, no less a person than the "king of tissue culturers," Prof. Alexis Carrel (1873–1944), Nobel prize winner in 1912, who acknowledged the existence of telepathy, clairvoyance, and miraculous cures, graphically said:

> *If we could visualise those immaterial links, human beings would assume new and strange aspects. Some would hardly extend beyond their anatomical limits. . . . Others would appear immense. They would expand in long tentacles attached to their family, to a group of friends, to an old homestead, to the sky and the mountains of their native country. Leaders of nations, great philanthropists, saints,*

would look like fairy-tale giants, spreading their multiple
arms over a country, a continent, the entire world.[184]

Distant Faith Healing

Therefore it is my opinion that *in the vast majority of such cures at a*
distance it is not the healer that heals but the expectant faith of the
patient!

I was intimately acquainted with the following instructive
case. A 66-year old political economist suffered a (repeated) severe concussion of the brain in an accident, which confined him
to his bed at the end of 1955. In mid-April 1956, he felt he was on
the danger list after the development of a phlegmon on the but-
tock (operated on successfully) followed by cystorrhea, pyelitis,
furuncle, and acataposis—the latter making it impossible for
him to take solid food. Since he did not sleep well either, the patient lost weight, going from 141 pounds to ca. 88 pounds. The
X-rays and the throat and stomach examination afforded no
clues. At this critical juncture, the patient pleaded with an occultist, who—so he said—had engaged in esoteric studies for
forty years, to surround him with healing thought-rays. Purely
out of compassion, the occultist agreed, and set times for the
evening transmissions although, privately, he was convinced
that this would not do much good to the sufferer who was plac-
ing such reliance on it.

What is more, pressure on his job meant that the "transmissions" could not be made daily, but only now and then. In spite
of this, the critically ill patient improved, became fit enough to
visit a spa house (where the atmosphere of the place cheered him
up), and got himself engaged to a nurse. *Not only he himself, but*
this nurse and others who were physically caring for him felt the "cur-
rent," for which he frequently expressed his thanks in writing;
and even a few days before his death on March 8, 1957 (following
another fall in December 1956 when taking a walk) he kept say-

---

[184]Carrel, Prof. Alexis, *Man, the Unknown* (London: Hamish Hamilton, 1935), p. 243.

ing, "The only one who really helped me at the time was Mr. X." Right up to the end, he always spoke of the healer with great gratitude and admiration.

This example is not an isolated one. "A student once asked Emile Coué (1857–1926) if he would think of him at a certain hour in order to help him *by thought-transference*. Some days later, the sufferer came to the class beaming and thanked Coué for the splendid result. Coué used to say with a mischievous smile that he happened to be with the angels at the appointed hour and completely forgot about the student." [185]

In April/May 1953, Dr. Hans REHDER, medical superintendent of a hospital for gastric diseases in Hamburg-Altona, wrote a personal account in "Hippokrates" of how he had arranged with a well-known spiritual healer that the latter would make remote thought transmissions to three critically ill female patients at set times. However, he did not tell the patients what he had done. The healer made the transmissions on three consecutive evenings from 9 o'clock through 9:15. Success: nil. Then REHDER undertook to lay a groundwork of faith. He told the three women stories of miraculous cures and said that now, on three consecutive days at stated hours, healing transmissions were going to be sent from a distance, and suggested that they might like to tune in to them inwardly. Yet (and this is the point) absolutely nothing was sent to them telepathically on the days in question! The result of this control experiment was that all three patients felt the "current," and one lady was cured of severe dropsy, a second of her jaundice, and the third, whose weight had fallen to 75 pounds after an operation on the pancreas, put on 33 pounds![186]

Nevertheless, even though this last example is certainly a model for much that goes on in so-called "spiritual healing," it is not necessarily the last word on the healer concerned. Subsequently, he wrote to me that in 1956 "energy changes in the organism of the sufferer" after distant treatment were measurable

---

[185]BRAUCHLE, Dr. Alfred, *Hypnose und Autosuggestion* [Hypnosis and Autosuggestion] (Leipzig, Reclams Univ. Bibl., No. 7208, 1936), pp. 24–25.
[186]HEGER, Gerhard, "Es gibt Wunderheilungen" [Miracle Cures Happen] in *Welt am Sonnabend* (1956), 20 [May 19]: 6; and Anonymous, "Durch den Glauben geheilt" [Faith Healing] in *Drogisten-Illustr.* (1958), January issue; REHDER, Dr. Hans, *Wunderheilungen* (Stuttgart: Hippokrates 1955), p. 19.

on the field-strength meter being developed by Dr. HAENSCHE, His desire to be objective does honor to this healer, and so does his opinion that the tests would need to be repeated a hundred times for exact proof.

EVIL SPELLS

When a medicine man curses a member of his tribe, an "old wizard" of a father mutters imprecations on his daughter, a witch ill-wishes a client who has refused to pay her,[187] or a mother—as the Stuttgart psychotherapist Dr. SOMMER only recently reported[188]—says to her small banana thief: "I hope it gives you a stomach-ache right now!" and sickness and death or "only" a colic are the result, these things are obviously the effects of autosuggestion primed by an insinuation from outside. It is not essential for the victim to hear the actual words when they are being spoken, it is enough for some meddlesome person to pass them on (as intended). But even if they are neither heard nor relayed, the idea that a powerful curse has probably been uttered is sufficient. One might say that this is the illegitimate counterpart of distant healing: *Maleficium in distans* [evil-doing from a distance].

Even Westerners give credence to black magic attacks. In Germany there are more people who believe they are being attacked by black magic "than are dreamt of in your philosophy."[189] Every so often we encounter requests for information on relevant protective measures in readers' letters sections of popular magazines, and there is hardly an "occult" author of repute who does not receive a despairing cry for help in the mail. Without doubt, there would be far more cases to add to the list if it were not for the fact that these people—like so many others who are obsessed—are afraid of being treated as mentally ill.

---

[187]MEMMINGER: p. 231.
[188]"Gibt es Heilung durch magische Kräfte?" [Is There Such a Thing as Healing by Magical Powers?] (Hamburg, 10-Pfg.-*Bild-Zeitung* 1958, 110 [May 13]: 2). (A same-day report from Stuttgart on a weekend conference of the Stuttgart Association of Physicians and Pastors).
[189]SHAKESPEARE, William, *Hamlet*, Act I, Scene 5 (first night in 1602, published in 1603).

GENUINE DISTANT HEALINGS

Whoever has had telepathic experiences is, in theory, able to perform telepathic healing. At the same time, it has to be pointed out that in telepathic therapy we are dealing with the transmission, not of abstract thoughts (although their transmission has been experimentally verified!), but of "ecstatic feelings" capable of relaxing the cramping and thus of healing the psychosomatic sufferer *directly*, or of taking part in the *indirect* healing of what are purely somatic diseases by relieving them, imparting a fresh stimulus, and banishing fevered thoughts.

But genuine distant healings are very rare. As has already been demonstrated, even the best deliberate "tuning-in" can activate the "receiver" in only a few instances. In other words, the number of genuine distant telepathic healings is infinitesimal. (The case is rather different where telepathic healings are performed at close quarters.)

Why is this? My own solution is that each individual is unique, and therefore so are the wave-lengths of his or her thoughts, as the Austrian cerebrologist, Dr. LEISBERGER, maintained as long ago as 1939. Nevertheless, close similarities undoubtedly exist between some individuals; for example, between identical twins.

Identical twins remain in especially close telepathic contact. Certainly in this case there is overwhelming evidence that compels us to postulate something in the nature of a telepathic-sympathetic connection. Identical twins often fall ill, meet with an accident, and die on the same day; yes, even at the same hour, of the same disease, or of the same external causes. Quite apart from the other shared factors in their destiny—since these can be seen as the results of inner disposition (the ratio of temperament to intellect) and of outer circumstances (because they look for the same things in their environment)—and apart from the similarity in their appearance and the agreement of their fingerprints, it is quite staggering to see how uniovular twins pursue a parallel path through life. They invariably have the same handwriting, fall ill at the same time, and, if criminally inclined, are brought to justice at the same time, even if superficially their life-styles are completely different! Those rare exceptions when there is a considerable gap between their times of birth only serve to prove the rule.* *The organic constitution of the two brains must be linked by approximately the same wave-lengths,* which express themselves in a similar type of modulation: so that the two individuals share a joint destiny.[190]

An analog occurs in so-called "plant-telepathy,"[191] celebrated in verse by no less a person than GOETHE:

When the vines come out in flower
The wine stirs in the vat.

What is more, LEISBERGER expressed the opinion that we must measure thought wave-lengths to work out which individuals are counterparts of one another. Possibly, before we are as advanced as this, *dactyloscopy,* which is a simpler method, could lend a helping hand. As a point of interest, it was used for identification purposes even in ancient China. The whorls on the finger-tips are unique to each individual, which explains the saying in ancient Pompeii: "He has left his thumb-print behind," as if to say that his personality has made an impression. The greater the similarity between the fingerprints of two persons, the easier and more certain—or at least so we may assume—is it for a bridge to be built between their thoughts.

In Chinese foundling-hospitals, the toeprints of anonymous newborn babies were recorded as soon as they were delivered, and so were the hair whorls on the crowns of their heads (in Chinese: *T'ou-ting-süanlo*). The whorl of hair and the brain-center underlying the whorl (the pineal gland) have played an important role in magic and mysticism, and possibly in telepathy, too.

---

*Astrologers would say that it is not so much the size of the gap between the two birth times that would make the twins less identical in many ways, but the arrival of a new Sign on the Ascendant between the times of their two births, whether that time was long or short. Of course, a big gap would be more likely to contain a change of Sign. *Translator's note.*

[190]HESSE, Reinhold, *Hellsehen auf naturwissenschaftlicher und allgemeinverständlicher Grundlage* [Clairvoyance Placed on a Scientific and Generally Intelligible Basis] (Hamburg, 1948), p. 12.

[191]KRÖNER, Dr. Walter, *Die Wiedergeburt des Magischen* [The Rebirth of the Magical] (Leipzig, 1938), p. 57; SCHRÖDTER, Willy, *A Rosicrucian Notebook* (York Beach, ME: Samuel Weiser, 1992), p. 8; and *Pflanzen-Geheimnisse* [Secrets of Plants] (Warpke-Billerbeck, 1957), p. 132 f.

TELEPATHIC CONNECTION BETWEEN BLOOD RELATIVES

Generally speaking, after identical twins, we would expect to find the most far-reaching (or rather "near-reaching") similarity of wave-lengths in blood relatives. And, in fact, instances of telepathic "SOS" calls, of telekinetic messages, and last, but not least, of shared emotions flashing through space between them are legion!

"Parents and children and children and parents are one body in two forms. Even though they are outwardly separate, they are still linked. The most secret thoughts pass from one to the other. Their sorrows have a reciprocal effect. They understand one another in their innermost being. Therefore they do not need words."[192] So said LÜ BU WE (died 232 B.C., Chancellor with the title "Second Father" under TSIN SCHI HUANG-DI [246–210 B.C.].

Here it seems appropriate to mention the "telepathy between mother and baby which is said to have been often observed. A mother who is breast-feeding begins to secrete milk as soon as the baby wants to drink, even when she and the child are not in the same place, and the mother has no way of knowing that the child is starting to feel thirsty at that very moment. Therefore the craving of the child must affect the mother by some agency that is not perceived by the five senses, and without her being aware of it, *before* lactation.

It is not being asserted that this will happen in every instance."[193] The editor of the journal in which this "short observation" appeared 70 years ago [i.e., in 1888], the traveler, colonial writer, and theosophist, Dr. Wilhelm HÜBBE-SCHLEIDEN (1846–1916), asked his lady readers to send accounts of experiences of the same sort. We do not know whether or not they did so; therefore we are repeating his request now.

While we are on the subject of "blood relatives," the following memorandum, which also appeared in various medical journals, is not without a certain interest:

---

[192]WILHELM, Richard, *Frühling und Herbst des Lü Bu We (Lü Schi Tschun Tsiu)* [The Spring and Fall of Lü Bu We (Jena, 1928), p. 115 f.
[193]HÜBBE-SCHLEIDEN, Wilhelm, "Telepathie zwischen Mutter und Säugling" [Telepathy between a Nursing Mother and Her Baby] in *Sphinx* (1888), 26 [February], 136 f.

The Manchester Guardian *reports that some three years ago veteran Frederick George Lee, who is now 34 years old, was asked by an employment agency if he would be willing to give blood for a 10-year old girl in the Middlesex hospital [in England]. Since then, Lee has given blood 25 times. In each of these operations, in which without exception the recovery depended on Lee's blood donation, he gave 36 pints. Usually the operations were successful, and today at least seventeen individuals owe their lives to Lee. For some time now he has been attached to the hospital as a "porter." He calls the recipients of his blood, his "blood relatives." Strange to say, although he could not have received any external notification of the fact, Lee has sometimes been aware of the death of a new "blood relative." "I feel severe pains in my arm and have to vomit," he said by way of explanation. He has repeatedly announced the exact hour of death. It should be noted that Lee is never—even during the operation—in direct contact with the patient. The blood is taken from him in another room.*[194]

Now the case of Lee, taken in conjunction with the well-authenticated injurious long-range emanation of *menstrual blood*,[195] can be produced as telling evidence for the reality of *"life* lights" (biolychnia) and "blood telegraphy."[196] In Hermetic circles (some of which are quite celebrated), the possibility of these things has been consistently rumored since Renaissance times. Seeing that "blood telegraphy," for example, was treated as a fact, in his instructions for using it, by the Martinist leader Dr. ENCAUSSE ("Papus") of Paris (who died in 1916 as a surgeon-major), it is timely and profitable to re-examine and throw fresh light on these old beliefs.

---

[194]ANONYMOUS, "Rätselhafte Folgen der Blutübertragung" [Puzzling Effects of Blood Transfusion], *Zbl. Okk* (1925), 6 [Dec.]: 2.
[195]SCHRÖDTER, Willy, *Geister/Mystik/Magie* [Spirits/Mysticism/Magic] (Berlin, 1958), pp. 117–120.
[196]SCHRÖDTER, Willy, *A Rosicrucian Notebook* (York Beach, ME: Samuel Weiser, 1992), p. 3 f.; 10 f.

Soulmates in Close Telepathic Contact

Quite often, soul affinity—or love—binds two people together more closely and securely than blood-relationship does. In 1952 a certain Professor RILLSTROEM (Upsala) allegedly demonstrated that the feeling of love between two persons is elicited by a so-far unknown form of radiation; which, incidentally, had already been postulated by the Callisoph, propounder of the new physiognomy and "helidopath" [*sic*, but see the reference to Huter's "helioda" below. *Tr.*] Carl HUTER![197]

Rillstroem's "Love Rays"

"As an organism, each individual emits rays of a certain wavelength. When two persons of the opposite sex but having the same (or, at least, nearly the same) wavelength meet one another, there springs up between them—with the consistency of a scientific law—love! The numerous individuals so far studied possess wavelengths between 0.085 and 1.542 millimeters."

The bringing together of two people by "undulatory selection" and the extremely high frequency of thought waves more or less falls in line with my own conjectures. However, highly desirable experimental proof has been denied me, because when I wrote to the above-mentioned investigator in August 1958 my letter was returned to me marked "unknown at this address." Since, unfortunately, my informant had not made a note of the source of the magazine article, I have been unable to pursue the matter.

Nevertheless, I have been gratified to learn that LHOTZKY'S "sympathy" and "antipathy," about which something will be

---

[197]HUTER, Carl, *Die Entdeckung der Lebensstrahlen: Die neue Heilwissenschaft*, Neuauflage. [The Discovery of Life Rays: The New Science of Healing. New Edition] (Althofnaß bei Breslau, 1932); BRANDT, G., *Carl Huters Helioda—die neuen Lebensstrahlen* [Carl Huter's Helioda—The Recently Discovered Life-Rays] (Detmold, 1907); KUPPER, Amandus, *Carl Huter und seine Forschungen im Lichte der Wahrheit. Eine Rechtfertigung.* [Carl Huter and His Researches in the Light of Truth. A Vindication] (Schwaig bei Nürnberg, 1924).

said later, reveal themselves in a rough-and-ready way as vibrations, which one day perhaps will be given a clear-cut scientific description. Today it is enough for us to note their reality. *In general, marriage depends on their existence."*

"Two Minds With But a Single Thought"

(The full quotation is: "Two minds with but a single thought, two hearts beating as one." It is taken from the end of Act II of *Der Sohn der Wildnis* [The Son of the Desert] [1842] by Friedrich HALM [Eligius Franz Joseph, Baron VON MÜNCH-BELLINGHAUSEN; 1806–1871]). Anyway, the notion that lovers' thoughts are literally "on the same wavelength" receives empirical backing from a whole stack of reports of telepathic cries for help, of presentiments, and above all of "shared feelings"!

Here is a very recent, striking example, which has been medically certified as true. A sufferer from *dementia paralytica* was being given the "malaria cure" in a Swiss mental institution a long way from home. His absent wife shared the inoculation-induced fevers psychogenically every time they occurred, even though the times of their occurrence were unknown to her.[198]

This illustrates the classic remark of the Marchioness DE SÉVIGNÉ (1626–1696) to her daughter Françoise-Marguerite, later the Countess DE GRIGNAN (1646–1705), who was racked by a chronic cough, "My child, I have pains in your chest."[199] What is more, the community of feeling between two individuals (French: *bipersonnalité*; Latin: *dipsychicum*) verifies a pronouncement of Marcus Portius CATO the Elder (234–149 B.C.): "The soul of a lover lives in a foreign body." This is so even when this "foreign body" happens to be of the same sex!

---

[198]FARNER, Dr. Gust., *Freiheit und Bindung in der Liebe* [Freedom and Bonding in Love] (Zürich, 1942), p. 42.
[199]TENHAEFF, p. 118.

"In 1760 Dr. Descottes treated in Argenton in the former Gouvernement Berry two young hysterical female lovers, one of whom knew what was happening to the other even when they were kept apart in separate houses." What is more, the two lesbians were "clairvoyants": "And she always foretold her own symptoms and those of her friend three or four days in advance."[200] Interesting as this is, we must avoid allowing ourselves to be side-tracked into a discussion of somnambulism at this point!

Sympsychicum—Polypsychismus (Egregor)

A temporary, cosy communion (or "common union") is created, for example, when lovers are strolling arm-in-arm, or young girls form a chain. Comfort is conveyed, confidence flows ("union is strength"), all hearts are beating in unison. The column of troops marching in step is welded into an "automaton" which has its counterpart in the army-worm or a cloud of gnats. The uniform movements and the monotonous intonation of certain formulas performed by the Islamic *Zikr* sect build up a temporary group-soul.[201] Freemasons of age and experience are said to be able to feel whether the invisible temple is well built or—because the "lodge spirit" is absent—is unstable.[202] However, the circle of fellow-creatures with whom one is capable of being in telepathic communication is relatively small, quite apart from the fact that a powerful stimulus may well be required for telepathy to take place. The bioclimatologist Dr. W. Werinos (Graz) says: "The wavelengths of the individual are tied to constitution and circumstances and can be altered by certain medicaments."[203]

(Also subject to influence is the luminosity of the human brain identified by De Crinis. It can be extinguished by chemical action.)

---

[200]Kluge: p. 295.
[201]Vett, Carl, *Seltsame Erlebnisse in einem Derwischkloster* [Strange Experiences in a Dervish Monastery] (Straßburg, 1931), pp. 97, 192.
[202]Ferger, N., *Mystik und Magie* [Mysticism and Magic] (Zürich, 1935), p. 180.
[203]Werinos, Dr. W., "Rätsel Schmetterling, Kristall" [Riddles, Butterfly, Crystal] Hamburg, 1956, 27 [end of October]f: 1115.

"Noxious Human Atmospheres"

We can now compare with these "certain medicaments" the "noxious human atmospheres" or psychogenic autotoxins which (as physiological accompaniments) precipitate very negative emotions in the various bodily humors. This condensation of "subsidiary excitation" (Charles Baudoin; born 1893) would provide a very satisfactory explanation of the fact that telepathic communication quite often occurs between individuals who are not intimately connected (due to an expansion of the wavelength width). The most virulent poison is produced by hatred, so it is not by chance that the previously mentioned masseuse in Baden-Baden was able to operate by active telepathy on the hated sanatorium patient, or that this frightened being (full of fear chemicals!) sensed the unheard and unseen comings and goings of her tormentor by passive telepathy. The hatred in the nurse was fuelled by envy,[204] which is a good sounding board for projecting one's emotions into another person.

Unusual Sensory Penetration

None other than Dr. August Wimmer (born 1872), Professor of Psychiatry at the University of Copenhagen and medical superintendent of the psychiatric-neurological hospital of the University, has given us a typical example: "Thus an unmarried lady suffering from senile dementia could perceive, in the form of sexual sensations, when her sister and brother-in-law (for whom she seemed to entertain warm feelings) were having sexual intercourse."[205]

Previously, Wimmer had related of a twenty-six year old patient in his ward that: "The empathy[206] exhibited by the patient, heightened as it was by his disease: his ability to assimilate other

---

[204]Hellberg, 90 f.
[205]Wimmer, Prof. August, "Über Besessenheit" [Possession], *Die okkulte Welt*, n.d., Bd. 135, p. 10 and footnote 14.
[206]Schrödter, Willy, "Einfühlung" [Empathy], *Neue Wiss.* (1957), 2 [Aug./Sept./Oct.]: 82–85.

persons and to feel their pains and movements, their heartbeats, urination and sexual responses, seemed positively medieval in its wizardry."[205]

Since envy was not a factor here, the empathy was not restricted to the sexual sphere as in the senile patient, and it was not focused on specific individuals, but was total and general; so WIM-MER was forced to exclaim: "This is possession of the finest water!"

"ECHO-SOUNDS" AND "PSYCHIC REFLEX WAVES" ("G-WAVES")

When a healthy person possesses the extremely rare faculty of high-grade empathy, and also has the necessary anatomical knowledge, he or she is in the position to make correct diagnoses amazingly often. Freelance engineer Demeter GEORGIEWITZ-WEITZER (SURYA; 1873–1949), who was absolutely impeccable" (according to SEBOTTENDORF) wrote concerning a lady who was a "passive-mantic" telepath of this sort, in a letter dated August 22, 1944 sent from Graz to a friend of mine, the lay medical practitioner Dr. Ernst BUSSE (born in 1893). The subject of his letter was the (former) naturopath Mrs. Käthe GÜNDL (born in 1881) of Vienna, who nowadays only makes diagnoses, and who, in 1941, was consulted by SURYA about an ear-complaint.

"This woman has a gift for making marvelous diagnoses in a few minutes. In order to do so, she sits *silently opposite* the patient, to whom she transmits certain "psychic waves." These are partly reflected and she then knows from the *reflex waves* what is wrong with the sick person. Now Mrs G. was rigorously examined for four weeks at the University Hospital in Vienna, ostensibly to find out if she could really make such superb diagnoses by ways not yet known to science. The professors issued the following pronouncement: "Mrs. Käthe GÜNDL indubitably possesses extraordinary diagnostic abilities, but as these cannot be explained scientifically, she must be forbidden to remain in practice." They knew, of course, that she had been a successful lay practitioner for thirty years!

---

[205] As last footnote but one.

In the illiberal climate of 1944, the "Thousand-year Reich"—whose own Führer was in fact possessed (for proof of this one need only recall his flabby, absent-looking, mediumistic face as photographed at the front line in 1914–1918!)—had a horror of people able to diagnose by their "physical radar system." It is to be hoped that, one day, the voluminous study (in progress since the end of the war) of this paragnostic diagnostician, who has so far been recognized only by private institutions, will yield a satisfactory scientific explanation of her skills.

We can now take a quick look at an "active-magic" counterpart of Mrs. GÜNDL, in the person of Dr. NEWTON (who died in the USA in 1895). On New Year's day in 1876, he succeeded in administering a "curative shock" to Dr. Franz HARTMANN, who was then in Texas; this was sufficient to free the latter individual from a weeping eczema "which had made his life a misery for 36 years."[207]

What is the source of such general telepathic abilities? My own explanation of these wide-ranging telepathic abilities, which permit their possessors—in contrast to the ordinary citizen—to make remote contact with anyone, is briefly as follows.

In every age a few individuals have given up what was merely a *persona* (Latin: "a mask"), ego, individuality, and desire for personal possessions and the "sin" of separation from their neighbors. Self-attachment is in fact a sin: not only does it segregate us from all other creatures, but it cuts our umbilical cord to the Centrum Centrorum [Center of Centers] and builds a dam between us and the impersonal ID. How close this is to "damnation"! As soon as someone has "depersonalized"[208] himself or herself in a moral sense, though not in the sense of surrendering thought and volition as a medium does (and then falls prey to vagrant influences), the ID—in accordance with the basic rule *Nequaquam vacuum*[209] fills him or her with its inexhaustible pow-

---

[207]HARTMANN, p. 146 (the chapter on "magical healing at a distance").

[208]Technical term used by Ricarda HUCH-CECONI (1864–1947) in the book *Entpersönlichung [Depersonalization]* (Leipzig, 1921).

[209]"A vacuum exists nowhere" [or, as we would say, "nature abhors a vacuum"]: axiom on the round altar tombstone of Christian Rosenkrantz in *Fama Fraternitas R.C.* (Cassel, 1614). [Issued in English in 1652 as *The Fame and Confession of the Fraternity of R: C: Commonly of the Rosie Cross*, reissued in facsimile with an introduction, by the Societas Rosicruciana in Anglia in 1923, also by Rudolf Steiner Publications, in *A Christian Rosenkrantz Anthology. Tr.*]

ers. The central "hook-up with the Absolute"[210] makes connections with every part of the Absolute: "If you dive deeply enough into your soul you will enter a region which is common to all living things. From there you can advance along the inner path to all that lives. . . . Now this whole, this commonality in the depths of your soul does not belong to you; on the contrary, you belong to it."[211] Carl Gustav JUNG (born in 1875) calls this lowest stratum "the Collective Unconscious." When people are linked by it, the phenomenon makes the "art of illusion" possible[212] as in the (Indian) instantaneous hypnosis of a crowd of spectators. Kirghizian shamans force an entry into the "deepest unconscious" (KOHNSTAMM) of another human being with the help of medicaments by using the confession poison *scorposkir*, which is obtained from scorpions (scorpion schnapps), for which purpose "it is important for the interrogator to take—an admittedly tiny— amount of the substance in order to form a link with the person under interrogation." The Russian scientist, Professor TELLMANN, who had fled to West Germany, revealed this in 1951.[213]

Dr. HÖSLI learned at first hand something about these "innermost powers of the unconscious." One winter's night, high up in the mountains, a young woman was almost on the point of death from postnatal hemorrhaging after what had been a fairly easy delivery. "Quite genuinely and in anguish of mind, one promised, one wished, to sacrifice one's own life if one could only save the mother for her baby. And a miracle occurred. It occurred not because of medical skill, but obviously because the fruit was not yet ripe enough to fall [her time had not yet come]. *Or did it perhaps occur because with one's inmost unconscious powers one was prepared to make a pact with death?*"[214]

However, let us remember a striking saying of the "Master of the Good Name," the Baal Shem Tov, Rabbi ISRAEL BEN ELIESER

---

[210]Technical term used by the philosopher Eduard VON HARTMANN (1842–1906) in his early work *Philosophie des Unbewußten* [Philosophy of the Unconscious] (1869).

[211]WIRZ, Otto, *Die geduckte Kraft* [The Servile Power] (Stuttgart, 1928), p. 185.

[212]SHCRÖDTER, Willy, *Geister/Magie/Mystik* [Spirits/Magic/Mysticism]. See the chapter on "The art of illusion," pp. 96–108; and "Hinduhypnotismus" [Hindu Hypnotism] made in Germany, *Mensch u. Schicksal* (1952), July 15: 9–11.

[213]SCHRÖDTER, Willy, Pflanzen-Geheimnisse [Plant Secrets] (Warpke-Billerbeck, 1957), p. 71; note 2.

[214]HÖSLI, 52.

(1700–1760), which, to modernize it a little, goes something like this: "Whoever wants to pray and be heard must be prepared to answer with his life before God for what he has requested."

Admittedly, this is where physics crosses the border into metaphysics, and the problem is lifted from the scientific plane onto the moral plane; but the inference that leads us to make this transition is, in my opinion, so persuasive, that it has to be drawn; it can well serve as a working hypothesis until some evidence is found to contradict it. What is operative here is the yoking (Indian *yoga*) of the Lower Ego (the desire nature) to the Higher Self.

The same thing was aptly put by the leading Theosophist and high-degree Mason, Hartmann with regard to the teachings of the *Mahatmas* (Indian: "great souls," or supermen, or masters), which were much in vogue in the circles in which he moved: "Whoever has learned to distinguish between his deathless 'I' and his transient personality, has found his master. He has become his own master, and his person is a disciple who is entrusted to him for training."[215]

Alchemy, like Hecate, was three-faced: it had metachemical-metallurgical (still to be discussed), physiological-macrobiotic, and spiritual-ethical aspects. In the technical language of *spiritual alchemy* in medieval Germany (a counterpart to Indian Yoga), the categorical imperative became: "Be ye transmuted from dead stones into living philosophical stones!"[216] That is to say, "You yourself must become the *lapis philosophorum*" (Latin for "stone of the wise") which, as a *panacea* (Greek for "all-healing"), bestows its *plusquamperfectum* on its neighbors. This perfection exists on all three planes. It is healing, it is morally uplifting, and it is restorative.

The same outlook was expressed in song years ago by the Rosicrucian-inclined "Silesian Nightingales" Angelus Silesius (III, p. 18):

---

[215]Hartmann, Dr. Franz, *Neue Lotusblüten* [Fresh Lotus Flowers], vol. I, (Leipzig,), p. 210.
[216]In imitation of I Peter 2: 5, the Frankfurt Paracelsist physician, Gerhard Dorn (Gerardu Dorneus) urges us: "Be transformed into living philosophical stones!" (*Spec. Phil. Theatr. Chem.* [1602]: I. p. 267). [See also, *Anima Magica Abscondita. The Works of Thomas Vaughan*, A.E. Waite, ed. (London: Theosophical Publishing House, 1919), p. 100. *Tr.*].

Enter into yourself
To find the Stone my friend,
And there will be no need
In foreign lands to wend.

Surely, the working hypothesis that exceptional abilities are associated with rare moral qualities is in keeping with the notion of
one universal moral order? Yet is "hypothesis" the right word to
use when we learn from the "varieties of religious experience"[217]
that such "charisms" (Greek: *charismen*, Indian: *siddhis*) are mile-
stones of inner development—though certainly not ends in
themselves—on the road to healing? This point is particularly
well made in the lapidary abstract prose of *The Yoga Aphorisms of
Patanjali*.[218]

    These basic ideas of the present work were put forward over
a quarter of a century ago in a study titled *Alchemy*, which con-
cludes that even the proximity of the "anointed" one, or coming
within the ambit of the latter's aura, is beneficial. The physician
is the physic. The physician's presence effects the cure. Here hallowing leads to healing—to being a healer in the proper sense of
the word (*Das Dritte Auge*, 1934, 12, 225).

OD AND TELEPATHY DO NOT EXPLAIN EVERY PHENOMENON

The three types of action discussed so far (odic, telepathic, and
mixed odic-telepathic) are insufficient to explain a whole series
of cases of an effect produced by pure presence!

    They do not really explain the everyday experience of the
sympathy or antipathy felt toward another person when we are
introduced to them ("first impressions"). As a rule, nothing odic

---

[217]Title of a book by William JAMES. Frequent reprints by Harvard University Press, Macmillan, Penguin, et al.
[218]OPPERMANN, Ing. M. A., *Die Yoga-Aphorismen des Patanjali* [The Yoga Aphorisms of Patan-jali] (Leipzig, ca. 1914; 1925); HAUER, Prof. Joh. Wilh., *Der Yoga als Heilweg* [Yoga as a Way of Healing] (Stuttgart, 1932); SCHMIDT, K. O., *Die Wissenschaft der Seele nach dem Yoga-Katchismus des Patanjali* [Soul Science According to the Yoga Catechism of Patanjali] (Pfullingen, 1922).

accompanies this sympathy or antipathy; that is to say, there is no projection or reception of a force that would immediately make the recipient of that force feel compatible or incompatible with its transmitter.

Again motivation by telepathy cannot be the answer when, on the occasion of a first encounter, there is a dismissive feeling (as often happens), even though it is apparent that all the other party wants to do is to meet us on neutral ground. Usually, if an attempt is made to create a good impression, the other person will pay close attention to body language, gestures, and speech. But it is not the way in which this person tries to present himself or herself that sinks into the bottom of our mind ("the ground of our soul"). No, something quite different moves us; which is the *cross-section of his or her being*, as I have said before. How this "distinct perception" is arrived at when the background reality is being deliberately hidden by the big parade in the foreground will be dealt with further on.

When, in 1911, Heinrich LHOTZKY (1859–1930) says of Madeleine *Bavent*, a character in a novel by the Polish Satanist and mystic Stanislaw PRZYBYSZEWSKI (1868–1927) that "merely by the atmosphere surrounding her she spread sins, orgies, and the witches' Sabbath in the convent,[219] when experience teaches that there do in fact exist such "high-power sexual transmitters" to whom men fly like moths to a candle-flame (the Blue Angel!), the matter cannot simply be one of Od, and the intensity of the influence is too great to be accounted for by telepathy alone.

But if there are those who can corrupt the morals of others by their presence, there must also be those who can do the reverse. For example, Lord LYTTON in his *Zanoni*, which he says is more than a romance, has delineated in the eponymous Chaldean adept a personality whose mere presence had a morally uplifting effect on "the sinners and publicans of the more polished world": "All appeared rapidly, yet insensibly to themselves, to awaken to purer thoughts and more regulated lives . . . nor . . .

---

[219]LHOTZKY, Heinrich, "Das Buch der Ehe" [The Marriage Book], (Königstein i.T. 1911), cited in v. SCHEFFER, Thassilo, *Philosophie der Ehe* [The Philosophy of Marriage] (Munich, 1944), p. 156.

did it seem that this change had been brought about by sober lectures or admonitions."[220]

In real life, Teddy LEGRAND stated the following in 1936 about the miracle healer THADDAEUS (Thaddée) in the Paris quarter of Plaisance: "When near him one felt indisputably better and mentally more alert—everyone agrees on this point."[221]

Once again the unsatisfactory nature of an explanation along the old accepted lines is clear. It is equally clear when, October 7, 1827, in the "Zum Bären" inn, GOETHE remarked in evening table-talk to his secretary Dr. Johann Peter ECKERMANN (1792–1854): "What is more, one psyche can elect to influence another by its mere silent presence, and I could relate several examples of this. For instance, I knew a man who—without uttering a word—suddenly silenced, by naked spiritual force, a company that had been full of animated conversation. Yes, he was able to inject a sense of unease, so that everything became miserable."[222]

I myself encountered a "wet-blanket" of this sort at a wedding in 1954. According to a press report in 1955, a Los Angeles barmaid could deliberately make her customers drowsy and unresisting, and they called her "naughty Susanne." The doubts of the Chasidic Tzaddikim were resolved in the presence of the founder of their sect, Rabbi ISRAEL BEN ELIESER (The Besht). Pilgrims streamed to the Bhagwan Sri RAMANA MAHARISHI (1879–1950) in Tiruvannamalai [sic Tr.] (South India) "not to see or hear anything, but in order to be able to meditate more easily than before in the atmosphere of a master, and also perhaps to be *irradiated by his illumination*."[223] When Julius EIGNER (Münstereifel) was silently irradiated with extra stamina by the hermit *Schwarzbart* ["Blackbeard"] in the Monastery of Internal Contemplation in the Huang-Shan mountains:

---

[220]LYTTON, Lord, *Zanoni* I. 6, pp. 96–97 (London: George Routledge & Sons, Ltd., n.d.).

[221]LEGRAND, Teddy, *Envouteurs, Guérisseurs et Mages* [Spellbinders, Healers, and Mages], (Paris, 1936), see the chapter, "The healer of Plaisance".

[222]ROSENBERGER, Ludw., *Geisterseher (nach Eckermanns "Gesprächen mit Goethe")* [Spiritists (After Eckermann's "Conversations with Goethe") (Munich, 1952), p. 46.

[223]VON VELTHEIM-OSTRAU, Dr. Hans-Hasso, *Der Atem Indiens* [The Spirit of India] (Hamburg, 1954), p. 256 f.

He said nothing more, but an unexpected power went out
from him; and after a while I felt it so strongly that I was no
longer able to follow my own thoughts. . . . Radiation of a rare
type came from him, an inexplicable force, which had no
equal.[224]

"It is said of Apollonius of Tyana (A.D. 10–97?) that *his silent*
arrival was all that was necessary to quell a riot."[225] In 1952, Prof.
Van Rijnberk discovered that, ". . . from human beings themselves, *without the need to do anything,* there radiates a perceptible
influence affecting the environment (*une action ambiante percepti-*
ble). Perhaps we should attribute to this radiation the fact that
some persons have emerged unscathed from revolutionary situ-
ations, and have even commanded respect from the upsurgents.
A case in point is that of "the unknown philosopher," Louis
Claude De Saint-Martin (1743–1803), who, although he was an
aristocrat and, as was common knowledge, kept in close contact
with the nobility—survived the storms of the French Revolution
without being harmed or molested."[226]

Marie Corelli (1864[?]–1924) in her semi-biographical romance of 1886 writes of an encounter with the young painter Raffaelo *Cellini* in Cannes:

While thus pacing about in feverish restlessness, I saw Cellini
approaching, his head bent as if in thought, and his hands
clasped behind his back. As he drew near me, he raised his
eyes—they were clear and darkly brilliant—he regarded me
steadfastly with a kindly smile. Then lifting his hat with a
graceful reverence peculiar to an Italian, he passed on, saying
no word. But the effect of his momentary presence upon me
was remarkable—it was electric. I was no longer agitated.
Calmed, soothed and almost happy I returned to Mrs. Ever-

---

[224]Eigner, Julius, *Gelbe Mitte—goldener Kreis* [Yellow Center—Golden Circle] (Hattingen
(Ruhr), 1951), pp. 279, 282.
[225]Surya, G. W., *Moderne Rosenkreuzer* [Modern Rosicrucians], (Pfullingen I.W., 1930), p. 73.
[226]Rijnberk, pp. 104–105.

ard, and entered into her plans for the day with so much alacrity that she was surprised and delighted.[227]

And when Cellini says of his first meeting with the Chaldean (Armenian) Count Casimir HELIOBAS, who incidentally was a real person:[228] "*. . . silently we walked side by side. A wonderful feeling of peace and relief had come over me—as great a relief as you my young lady—so I have observed—experience when in my company.*"[229] And on May 12, 1890, VON NUSSBAUM (1829–1890), in the capacity of an expert witness, declared on oath that: "There are certain people who have a very soothing effect, and there are others who have the opposite."[230]

With regard to animals, it is repeatedly said of some horse-breakers, real and fictional, that they are able to tame any horse without resorting to professional tricks—even though they are quite unable to say how they do it.[231]

With regard to plants, there are "certain plants that respond badly to people who emit a harmful radiation. If a person of this sort approaches or even handles them, these plants exhibit every sign of agitation, faintness, and collapse. In rooms that are full of an evil human *aura* they wilt and die. If they are worn as a button-hole by individuals who are detrimental to them, it is amazing how quickly they lose their scent and beauty, how soon they droop and wither."[232]

On one occasion, STERNEDER saw with his own eyes how all the daisy flowers rapidly turned away from someone well

---

[227]CORELLI, *Romance* I, pp. 9–10.
[228]SURYA, G. W. and STRAUSS, Dr. Alfr., *Theurgische Heilmethoden* [Theurgic Methods of Treatment] (Lorch i.W., 1936), p. 221.
[229]CORELLI, p. 76.
[230]GRATZINGER, p. 5 f.
[231]LERNET-HOLENIA, Alexander, *Die Frau im Zobel* [The Woman in Sable] (Munich, 1954) (List-Buch No. 32), p. 37; DU PREL, Dr. Carl, *Die Entdeckung der Seele durch die Geheimwissenschaften* [The Discovery of the Soul through the Occult Sciences] vol. II (Leipzig, 1895), p. 236; SCHRÖDTER, *Offenbarungen* [Revelations] (Fall Ezer), p. 11; RIKO, A. J., *Handbuch zur Ausübung des Magnetismus, des Hypnotismus, der Suggestion, der Biologie und verwandter Fächer* [A Practical Handbook of Magnetism, Hypnotism, Suggestion, Biology and Related Subjects] (Leipzig, 1904), p. 129 f.
[232]HUEBNER, Dr. Friedr. Markus, *Menschen als Arznei und Gift* [People as Medicines and Poisons] (Kampen/Sylt, 1934), p. 38.

known in Gloggnitz as a drunkard, liar, and ill-treater of animals. They turned to face the east, even though the summer sun was shining brightly in the south."[233] "Besides they say if the flower withers she wears she's a flirt." [James JOYCE][234]

With regard to inanimate objects, "letters convey atmospheres, and those who are sensitive to such things can read between the lines."[235]

Letters have an immediate salutary effect on the body, as I myself experienced in December 1940 on receiving a letter from Surya. On letting him know, I had the following reply dated December 7: "This is nothing new to me because I am constantly receiving similar reports from friends and those who are ill. As soon as the latter have opened and read my letters, there has been a marked improvement in their condition (even in the case of children who have not themselves read the letters but have had them read to them by their parents) and *they have recovered without medicine from that same hour . . .*"

---

[233]STERNEDER, *Sommer* [Summer], p. 67.
[234]JOYCE, *Ulysses* vol. II (Bodley Head, 1960), p. 481.
[235]DRESSER, p. 40.

PSYCHOGENIC AUTOINTOXICATION

We must always bear in mind the possibility of poisoning by animal fluids produced by anger!
—*Dr. Ernst v.* FEUCHTERSLEBEN[236]

In the psychology laboratory of the University of Washington in 1879, the "psychurg" Elmer GATES (1859–1923) professor of psychology at the Pennsylvania School of Industrial Art obtained experimental proof for the traditional belief that negative emotions embitter people, making them ill and full of gall. (*Anima enim nequam disperdet qui se habet* [A wicked soul shall destroy him that hath it] Sirach VI, 4). He asked a number of test subjects to breathe into frozen glass tubes, and added rhodopsin iodide (visual purple) to the precipitate. In those who were in a placid frame of mind, the mixture did change its appearance, but in those who were under an emotional strain, colored sediments were deposited; for example, they were gray in grief and depression, pink in remorse, and brown in anger. This clearly indicated that chemical changes had taken place in the volatile substances contained in the breath. If these condensates were injected into other individuals, the emotional states of those who had breathed them out were passed on to them.

Jealousy liquid given to a guinea-pig by intravenous injection killed the animal within a few minutes. Hatred is the strongest emotional poison. Enough corrosive hatred can be exhaled in an hour to kill four strong men. As already mentioned, a "burning hatred" will cause lupus. An illness due to emotional causes (the *Ens Astrale* of PARACELSUS) cannot be eradicated by material remedies; the first thing to do is to eradicate the causes

---

[236]VON FEUCHTERSLEBEN, Baron Ernst, *Zur Diätetik der Seele*, ed. Gesenius (Halle/S. 1910), p. 71, footnote, 1838.

by a change of heart. Following that, material aids are often unnecessary, although they might help to speed recovery as sup-
plements.[178] Similar results are said to have been obtained by
Bulgarian researchers when running tests on examination candi-
dates and on invalids. Positive emotions created beneficial
chemical reactions in the human body. More than 40 good reactions and a similar number of bad ones were discovered in the
perspiration and secretions of the individuals concerned.[237] Yogis
and black magicians have known from time immemorial about
poison-forming stimuli,[238] and even in antiquity the latter have
used precipitates obtained by nefarious practices. In fact, I have
all the relevant details, but do not think it would be wise to pub-
lish them. Instead of doing so, I would suggest (to take a hint
from blood banks) that the breath fluids of peaceful and kindly
individuals should be stored for use on people who are dis-
turbed, tormented, anxious, and debilitated. The "father of medicine," HIPPOCRATES of Cos (460–377 B.C.), knew, even in his day,
that "anger and fear generate a poison in the body," and
Friedrich VON SCHILLER (1759–1805) put the following monologue
into the mouth of his *Wilhelm Tell* (1804): "You have changed the
milk of pious thoughts for me into fermenting dragon's venom"
[4, 3].

Everyday experience forcibly draws our attention to the fact
that negative emotions do indeed poison the milk that ought to
soothe and pacify. The baby brings it up in a spasm! It is as un-
palatable to the child as venison from a deer that has been
hunted to death is to adults, because its death throes have
brought about organic changes in the animal.[239]

As we have already seen, mental emotions are precipitated
not only in the breath, but also in the perspiration and secretions.
It is not only the bite of a mad dog that is deadly: it was reported
in England some years ago that one sister had bitten another in a
fit of temper and the one who had been attacked died within

---

[178]See earlier footnote, page 60.

[237]RIEDLIN, p. 49; DUNBAR, F. L., VON KALCKREUTH, *Von tausend Dingen* [A Thousand Things]
(Leipzig, 1937), p. 42; WACHTELBORN, Karl, *Die Heilkunde auf energetischer Grundlage und das
Gesetz der Seuchen* [Medical Science Based on Energetics and the Law of Contagion]
(Hellerau-Dresden, 1940), I, p. 289 f.

[238]KERNEIZ, C., *Der Hatha-Yoga* [Hatha Yoga] (München-Planegg, 1938), p. 217.

[239]JAEGER, Gustav, *Die Entdeckung der Seele* [The Discovery of the Psyche] (Leipzig, 1880).

three days. Be that as it may, the bite of someone belonging to a foreign race can produce dangerous abscesses.[240] And it is a known fact that saliva can undergo a sudden chemical change, as evidenced by a bitter taste. On the other hand, homeopathy removes the harmful effect of negative emotions with the bitter remedy *Ignatia*.[241] In the C 30 potency it acts "instantaneously" when the leading symptoms are "quiet grief and melancholy."[242]

It is a popular opinion, which I happen to share, that chronic negative moods, or ill-humors, damage the heart. PYTHAGORAS (580–493 B.C.) advises: "Do not eat your heart out!" Which is something that modern business executives would do well to heed.[243] Chinese clinical diagnosis is in agreement: "The heart of a patient partial to bitter things is unhealthy."[244] On the other hand, there is a saying in Germany that "what is bitter in the mouth is good for the heart," which suggests a recognition of the possibility of "taste therapy" as practiced in Tibet.[245] If psychological emotions were not precipitated physically and chemically, it would not be possible to treat them homeopathically.[246] Thus, Dr. Arthur LUTZE (1813–1870) treated them successfully with high potencies (D 30). Anyway, in his latter years, "old Lutze" saw in bio-magnetism the primary agent in the homeopathic remedies he manufactured personally by manual succussion![247]

When a change in the chemical composition of the breath is brought about by the emotions, this occurs through the meeting

---

[240]KARLIN, Alma M., *Der Todesdorn* [The Sting of Death] (Berlin, 1931), p. 281.

[241]SURYA, G. W., *Schlangenbiß und Tollwut* [Snakebite and Rabies] (Lorch I. W., 1929), p. 40.

[242]WIENER, Kurt, "Die leidigen Hochpotenzen" [The Troublesome High Potencies] *Allg. hom. Ztg.* (1956), 3: 90–96. Reported in: "Die Wirksamkeit homöopathischer Hochpotenzen" [The Effectiveness of Homeopathic High Potencies] *Erfahr.hk.* (1956), 8 [August]:388. [See also: *The Magic of the Minimum Dose.*, Dr. Dorothy Shepherd (London: Homæopathic Publishing Co. 1938 and later editions). A homeopathic classic and very readable! *Tr.*].

[243]SCHRÖDTER, Willy, "Die Herren der Zeit" [The Time Lords] *Okk. Stimme* (1953), 25 [February]: 19 f.

[244]FRICHET, p. 60.

[245]BADMAJEFF, Dr. Wladimir, *Chi-Schara-Badahan: Grundzüge der tibetanischen Medizin* [The Chief Features of Tibetan medicine] (Pfullingen i.W. n.d., ca. 1920); VON KORVIN-KRASINSKI, P. Cyrill, *Tibetische Medizinphilosophie* [Tibetan Medical Philosophy] (Zürich, 1953).

[246]GALLAVARDIN, Dr. Jean-Pierre, *Homöopathische Beeinflussung von Charakter, Trunksucht und Sexualtrieb* [Homeopathic Influencing of Character, Alcoholism, and Sexuality] (revised by Dr. Hans TRIEBEL (Ulm/Donau; Karl F. Haug Verlag, 1958).

[247]SURYA, G. W., *Homöopathie, Isopathie, Biochemie, Iatrochemie und Elektrohomöopathie* [Homeopathy, Isopathy, Biochemistry, Iatrochemistry, and Electrohomeopathy] (Berlin-Pankow, 1923). pp. 101–103.

of air and blood in the filter tissue of the lungs. Therefore it is the blood that is primarily impregnated, and it passes on this impregnation to the breath second hand. "Salus"-MÜLLER ascertained that "an energy is present in the human body that emerges with the breath and more especially from the fingertips and is similar in effect to radioactivity.[248]

Dr. Albert CAAN, former First Assistant at the Heidelberg Institute for Cancer Research, announced, in 1911, that tests had shown that human organs that have never been in contact with radium do, nevertheless, contain a radioactive substance of their own, which possesses the ability to make the air a conductor.[249]

And thus, we might add, a suitable vehicle for the transmission of "psychoelectric thought waves."[250] Dr. H. LANGBEIN (Niederlößnitz/Sa.) "tried to give a scientific explanation of the paths traced by the pendulum" in terms of human radioactivity.[251] Blood may be magnetized,[252] but cannot be used as a vehicle with which to magnetize. However, its assistant, the breath, can certainly be used in this way, by means of the technique known as "adspiration," formerly insufflation, both of which were called a "transfusion vitale" by Professor Hector DURVILLE (1849–1923) of Paris, in a brochure of the same name, on account of their long-known use *in extremis*.[253] The inclusion of "Pfeiffer's crystallization diagnosis"[254] in the "Gates experiment" would probably produce the most interesting results.

---

[248]MÜLLER, E. K., p. 31.

[249]CAAN, Dr. Albert, *Über Radioaktivität menschlicher Organe* [Radioactivity of Human Organs], Heidelberger akad. Ber., 5 Abhdlg. (Heidelberg, 1911); GÄDICKE, p. 74; GESSMANN, G. W., *Aus übersinnlicher Sphäre* [From the Supernatural Sphere], (Leipzig and Vienna, 1921), p. 150.

[250]PAULK-KEMSKI, E., "Was ist Psychokratie?" [What is Psychocraty?] *Prana-Bibliothek* No. 8), p. 8. (Leipzig n.d.).

[251]LANGBEIN, Dr. H., *Die Pendelbahnen und ihre wissenschaftliche Aufklärung durch Radioaktivität* [Pendulm Gyrations and Their Scientific Explanation through Radioactivity] (Diessen vor München [Munich], 1914), p. 14.

[252]THETTER, pp. 236–237.

[253]KLUGE, p. 321 f.

[254]PFEIFFER, Dr. Ehrenfried, *Empfindliche Kristallisationsvorgänge als Nachweis von Formungskräften im Blut* [Sensitive Crystallization Processes as Evidence of Formative Forces in the Blood] (Dresden, 1936); SELAWRY, A. and O., *Die Kupferchlorid-Kristallisation* [Copper Chloride Crystallization] (Stuttgart, 1956); KRÜGER, Hans, *Kupferchlorid-Kristallisationen, ein Reagenz auf Bildekräfte des Lebendigen* [Copper Chloride Crystallizations, a Reagent for the Formative Forces of Living Creatures].

Blood Emanation is Easier to Impregnate than Blood

But if such important substances belonging to the physical body—and we are thinking in particular of the blood, of which Moses (ca. 1225 B.C.) who had been adopted by Pharaoh's daughter Thermutis, and was "learned in all the wisdom of the Egyptians"[255] plainly stated, "the blood is the life" [NEPHESH][256]—how much stronger and long-lasting must the influence be on that subtle fluid essence for which "Salus"-MÜLLER gave the objective electrical evidence that it is "undoubtedly an emanation of the blood."[257]

Control of the Blood-Flow: "Tumo," "Ilm el Miftach," Kerning

At this point, I wish to make a short digression, for "I am unwilling to trim a thought as soon as it acquires breadth and freedom."[258] Thus: "MÜLLER was able to supply proof that this emanation was emitted with the breath and more especially by the fingertips, and displayed an effect similar to radioactivity."[259] MÜLLER himself found that: "Apparently the intensity of the emanation gradually changes according to the amount of blood momentarily present in the emission region concerned and on the closeness of the blood to the surface of the body."[260]

As intimated in my *Grenzwissenschaftlichen Versuchen*[36] [Parapsychological Experiments], one of the main "psychological exercises" widely publicized by the New Thought movement at the turn of the century was the so-called "control of the blood."[261] It consisted (with or without the help of a suggestion formula) of

---

[255] Acts 7: 22.
[256] Deuteronomy 12: 23.
[257] MÜLLER, E. K., p. 31, sub. 2.
[258] SCHENK, Gustav, *Schatten der Nacht* [Shadow of the night] (Hanover, 1939), p. 56.
[259] RINGGER, Dr. Peter, *Parapsychologie* [Parapsychology] (Zürich, 1957), p. 67.
[260] MÜLLER, E. K., p. 31, sub 3.
[36] As earlier footnote, page 14.
[261] ERTL, Hans, *Vollständiger Lehrkurs des Hypnotismus etc.* [A Complete Course of Instruction in Hypnotism], 7th ed. (Leipzig, n.d.), pp. 83–84.

concentrating one's attention on some part of the body and, if applicable, keeping the latter still at the same time.[262] What was attempted—quite often with some success—was to tone up the muscles and to warm cold hands and feet. On the latter point it is interesting that SCHULTZ,[263] the deviser of "Autogenic Training" "has measured a rise in temperature of radiated body heat of more than 1° C" during the "warmth exercise," that is to say, during concentration on an arm in the mental expectation that it would become quite hot. The psychologist Dr. A. SEVERIN (Cologne) reported that by fixing the gaze on a hand held horizontally at eye-level, and by repeating aloud a suggestion formula to the effect that the hand would become warmer, test subjects could obtain a temperature difference between their two hands of up to 4° C.[264] The Tibetan *Respa* masters with their similarly based *tumo*, keep themselves warm, even without clothing, on the icy plateaus in winter; for which reason they call these exercises the "soft warm mantle of the gods."[265]

Islamic esotericism (*Tarikaat*) has known since the days of MUHAMMAD (KUTDAM IBN ABDALLAH; 570–632) a secret training called *Ilm el miftach* (science of the key) or *Ilm el nizan* (science of balance). It consists of "considering" (and fixing one's eyes on) the vertically raised index finger and the thumb stuck out at right angles, while internally spelling out certain words from the *Koran*. Naturally this *modus procedendi* also results in a sensation of heat; but its object is to strengthen the biomagnetism, and this is said to bring about a consolidation and emancipation of the "meta-organism" (Lazar von HELLENBACH-CHECH; 1827–1887).[266] Jacques COEUR (1395–1456), the counsellor and financier of King CHARLES VII of France (1422–1461) nicknamed "The Victorious" (also "The Well-Served") owned a house that still stands in

---

[262]BONDEGGER, H. W., *In zwei Stunden nicht mehr nervös?* [Cured of Nerves Within Two Hours?] (Dresden: Talisman-Bücherei, 1936), pp. 49–50.

[263]SCHULTZ, J. H., *Übungsheft für das Autogene Training* [Autogenic Training Workbook] (Leipzig, 1935), p. 18.

[264]SEVERIN, Dr. A., "Die Autosuggestion, etc." [Autosuggestion etc.], *Neugeistbuch No. 27*, p. 17, Pfullingen n.d. (ca. 1918).

[265]DAVID-NEEL, pp. 212, 214 f., 218–223, 225.

[266]v. SEBOTTENDORF, Baron Rud., *Die Praxis der alten türkischen Freimaurerei* [The practice of Old Turkish Freemasonry] (Leipzig, 1924), p. 39; (Freiburg i.B., 1954), p. 44.

Bourges (Cher), and is decorated by two towers that remind one of a thumb and finger.[267]

Staring at the index finger gradually induces the smell of sulfur, then the taste of mercury sublimate, and finally the taste of salt.[268] Owing to these chemical-physiological changes, this hermetic discipline is also spoken of as *Ilm el quimija* (the science of chemistry). The smell of sulfur is typical of a strong increase in magnetic force. Around A.D. 900, Arabic esoteric knowledge was picked up by the wide-awake Venetians, and later on in Germany it formed the basis of a system of physiological alchemy. The Rosicrucians treated it as a "hidden secret" which might be represented only in pictures.[269]

The hand positions of Turkish Freemasonry are occasionally depicted in the images of saints in old churches. Thus in September 1958, I ascertained that the parish church of Pürgg (Ennstal) dedicated on St. Alexius' Day (July 17) in 1130 by the bishop of Gurk (HILTEBOLD; 1106–1131) housed two of these: Zacharias, shown [incorrectly] in the robes of a high-priest with the breastplate (containing the "Urim and Thummim"), forms the letter "O" with his left hand, and Elizabeth (his wife) makes a "breast grip" in the form of the letter "A." There is a charnel house in the church, which has given it a local reputation of being haunted. Behind the little church rises the mighty Grimming (7546 ft.), which Rome's legionaries regarded as *mons altissimus Styriae* [the highest mountain in Styria], which demands an annual sacrifice and has a seeming door on its south side. Paula GROGGER (born in 1892) wrote about this in the powerful, Styrian, regional novel *Das Grimmingtor* [The Grimming Door] (1926). A modern offshoot is the "letter exercises" of J. B. KERNING (Joh. Bapt. KREBS; 1774–1851), the so-called "Kerning Mystic" [Kerning's system differentiates between "mysticism" and "mystic." See WEINFURTER'S book refer-

---

[267]v. SEBOTTENDORF, Leipzig, p. 24; Freiburg i. B., p. 29; HEYM, Gérard, *L'étrange destin de Jacques Coeur* [The Strange Fate of Jacques Coeur] (Nîmes, 1953); CANSELLIET, Eugène, *Jacques Coeur (La Tour Saint Jacques)* [Jacques Coeur (The St. James Tower)] (1957), 8 [Jan./Feb.]: 73–82.
[268]v. SEBOTTENDORF, Leipzig, 1924, pp. 15, 36; Freiburg i.B., 1954, pp. 19 f., 42.
[269]SCHRÖDTER, Willy, *Geschichte und Lehren der Rosenkreuzer* [The History and Doctrines of the Rosicrucians] (Villach, 1956), pp. 119–124; and *A Rosicrucian Notebook* (York Beach, ME: Samuel Weiser, 1992), pp. 78f., 250f.

enced below. *Tr.*][270] The source of all these doctrines is the age-old *Kundalini Yoga* of Indian Tantra.[271]

ENGRAMS IN THE OD

The "Gates effect" is elicited not only by non-recurring, powerful, *active* emotions (if we may call them that), or, to put it another way, by a state of *exaltation*, which incidentally does not last long (sudden anger being one example), but also by suppressed, *quasi-passive* emotions, associated with a depressive state. In the latter, the length of the exposure time offsets a brief maximum intensity, although Dr. Gustav RIEDLIN[272] alleges that "deep grief over the death of a child expressed itself by a gray coloration in the fluids," and grief is a long-lasting emotion. It seems safe to assume that the same applies *mutatis mutandis* [when the requisite changes are made] to positive moods: here a sudden surge of great joy, and there a state of satisfaction in which "seeking and finding" the innermost heart (Japanese: *hara*) is reached. Possibly the *Tawara nodes* also known as *Aschoff-Tawara* nodes are associated with these emotions.[273]

These "vestibular nodes" in the heart, which form part of its conduction system, were discovered by the Japanese anatomist Sunao TAWARA (born in 1873). We have already said, of course, that all *emotionally toned thinking* (and it is only our feelings that are alive, thinking being but a twiglet on the "golden tree"), in both the positive and negative sense, must express itself and its imaginations more clearly in the plastic Od than in any other ma-

---

[270]KERNING, J. B., *Briefe über die Königliche Kunst* [Letters on the Royal Art] (Lorch i. W., 1912); STRAUSS, Dr. Alfr. & SURYA, G. W., *Theurgische Heilmethoden* [Theurgic Healing Methods] 2nd ed., p. 185 f.; SCHRÖDTER, Willy, "Hautmediumität" [Skin Mediumship], *Mensch und Schicksal* (1955), 21 [January 15]: 8 f.; DORNSEIFF, Franz, *Das Alphabet in Mystik und Magie* [The Alphabet in Mysticism and Magic] (Berlin, 1922), pp. 152–153.
[271]WEINFURTER, Karl, *Der brennende Busch* [The Burning Bush] (Lorch i.W., 1930); ROUSELLE, Dr. Erwin, "Seelische Führung in lebendigen Taoismus" [A Spiritual Introduction to Living Taoism], *Eranos-Jb.* (1933), pp. 169, 184.
[272]RIEDLIN, p. 49.
[273]WETTERER, Frz. Jos., *Das Wesen der Seele* [The Nature of the Psyche] (Engen/Hegau, 1949).

terial, but the statement bears repeating here because of what we have to say next.

What is called "emotionally-toned thinking" includes life-long character traits of the individual, such as anxiety, a love of money, pride, power-hunger, or a search for sexual conquests on the negative side, and striving for justice ("not able to stand idly by while any injustice is being done"), and innate kindness on the positive side.

As I remarked at the beginning of my exposition: what impresses the unprejudiced mind when we first meet people is their cross section, the "characterological balance" of the life they have lived so far. That is to say, we see people as they are—and what they are is as they "think in their heart"—and not as they present themselves and would like to be seen. The Jewish secret doctrine known as the Kabbalah (literally, "tradition") puts it this way: "Behind the will stands the wish"; which means that behind the deliberately assumed mask lie the propensities. And it is this true state of affairs (projecting itself from the unconscious) that speaks to us. The mask—which is a product of conscious abstract thought—makes little impression on us. Finally, as far as the "mixed types" are concerned, it is what obeys the inner voice that speaks to us; it carries more weight than what has been worked up afterward for presentation. However, both make some impression!

OD IS NOT OD

At this point we need to realize that Od is not simply Od! Not only is odic supercharging—which can be achieved through various techniques (such as controlling the circulation of the blood, Laya-Yoga, or the Indian science of breath known as Pranayama) or even, temporarily, by stimulants such as alcohol[274]—evidence enough, but even more convincing proof lies in *Od torment*. And that is quite independent of the moral qualities of its transition stage!

---

[274]MÜLLER, E. K., p. 31; NIELSEN, S. 151 f.

Surely it would be quite wrong to assume that physical healing powers are all the healer needs. I had a professional colleague
in Munich, colonial director (Alfred) Wilhelm SELLIN (1841–1933)
who died at age 91 ten years ago. He became a writer after his re-
tirement, and as a sideline, he treated free of charge thirty sick
people every day until he reached age 88. He himself lived in the
most straitened circumstances. The deceased was an extraordinarily high-minded personality, possessing rare psychical and
spiritual gifts. He was constantly referring to the development of
psychic and spiritual healing powers, and substantiated their existence as follows: "You don't imagine do you," said he, "that
these healing life forces are just to do with physical virility? Here
comes a hefty young fellow as tall as a tree for treatment. He
could put two old-timers like me in his pocket, and yet I cure him
of his severe bronchitis."[275]

Let Hector DURVILLE speak for the many others who share
the opinion that: "The animal magnetism in the human body is
actually determined by the moral type of the individual."

On the same lines, professor of agriculture Oskar KORSCHELT
(1841–?), the inventor of apparatus for the collection of cosmic
forces ("solar etheric radiation apparatus") as a partial substitute
for *animal magnetism*, considered the possibility of a mutual infection of character being brought about by magnetizing (formerly called, appropriately enough, *Neurogamy*; Greek for "nerve
marriage"!): "It is not only the life force, but also the character, of
the healer that is shared with the sick person. Conversely, the
character of the patient flows into the healer."[276]

---

[275]THETTER, p. 62 f.; In the first edition of his book, which came out in Mährisch-Ostrau in
the early 40s, we read "who died some years ago at age 91." I have officially investigated
the discrepency in the dates and have discovered that SELLIN was born on July 10, 1841, and
died on September 10, 1933; the cremation took place in Munich on September 14, 1933.
[276]KORSCHELT, Prof. Oskar, *Die Nutzbarmachung der lebendigen Kraft des Äthers in der
Heilkunst, Landwirtschaft und Technik* [The Utilization of the Living Force of Ether in Medicine, Agriculture and Technics] (Bad Schmiedeberg, u. Leipzig, n.d., ca. 1891), p. 72;
KALLENBERG, Friedr., *Offenbarungen des siderischen Pendels* [Revelations of the Sidereal Pen-
dulum], (Diessen, 1921), p. 31; DURVILLE, Hector, *Die Physik des Animal-Magnetismus (Ani-
mismus)* [The Physics of Animal Magnetism] (Leipzig, 1912), p. 26.

AURA

The definiteness of the anatomical contours is partly an illusion. Each one of us is certainly larger and more diffuse than his body.

—*Prof. Alexis* CARREL, *M.D.* [184]

Od does not end at the surface of the skin. It extends beyond the contours of the physical frame and envelops it, like a second fine body "flaming out" of it. This is the *aura* (Greek: "breeze"; a similar-sounding word in Hebrew is 'or = "light," and metaphorically the "light of life"). Usually it is invisible to human eyes unless it is exceptionally intense and therefore massive, as it is in the case of saints for example. The so-called *halo* is a fact! Major Francis YEATS-BROWN has "very often observed that the skin of a *guru* (Indian, "teacher," "guide") began to shine in the dark."[277] The *Yoga Sutras of Patanjali* promise the halo through a special breathing exercise (*pranayama*): "effulgence by mastery over *samâna*" (III; 40). The circle of light around the skin of the saints is known as a *nimbus* or *gloriole*, that around the whole body is called an *aureole* or *glory*, or a *mandorla* (Italian, "almond") when stylized as an oval. By *xénologues* it is sometimes called the "auric egg." But even in ordinary persons, especially if they are overexcited or hysterical, the shining of the body can be seen by people with normal vision (non-sensitives).[278] Radiation of normal intensity lying in the wider spectrum, is perceived directly only by *sensitives* (clairvoyants). For a high percentage of those with normal vision, Dr.

---

[184]See earlier footnote, page 64.
[277]YEATS-BROWN, Francis, *Ist Yoga für dich?* [Is Yoga for You?] (Berlin, n.d.), p. 169.
[278]ORTT, Felix, "Die menschliche Aura" [The Human Aura], *Zbl. Okk.* (1926), December issue: 267 f.

Walter J. KILNER, M.R.C.P. (London) made the aura visible with his "Kilner screens" or "dicyanin screens."[279]

Oscar BAGNALL developed an improved product known as "auraspecs" or "Kilner goggles."[280] An image is impressed on a photographic plate that has been exposed to the aura.[281] In other words, the aura has been actually photographed.[282] The Russian Privy Counsellor, Jakob VON NARKIEWICZ-JODKO photographed radiations from the hands at the turn of the century: in the case of sympathy (the hands of a bride and bridegroom) there was a lively interchange of Od between the upper extremities when they were held a few centimeters away from one another; where antipathy held sway, the emanating Od formed an unmistakable mark of separation.[283] He called his process "Electrography." When Ernst SCHÄFER (born in 1911) in Lhasa on his Tibetan expedition of 1938–1939 frequently photographed the aura round the *Gyalpo*, or regent, Reting HUTUKTU, painstakingly and with a variety of apparatus, the other persons in the picture were in sharp focus, but the image of the spiritual dignitary was unrecognizable, hazy, and decomposed into streaks!

"It became clear to SCHÄFER that a special phenomenon must be present; so he referred the matter to a well-known expert in the psychology of religion, Dr. Eberhard COLD. The latter came to the following conclusion: 'What you have filmed is the typical phenomenon of the *aureole, and this was emanating from the whole body of the king.*'"[284]

A similar case is that of a young Jewish refugee from Germany investigated by VAN RIJNBERK in 1939 in the physiological

[279]KILNER, Walt. J., *The Human Atmosphere or the Aura Made Visible by the Aid of Chemical Screens* (London, 1911). [Kilner's book: *The Human Atmosphere (The Aura)*, first edition published September, 1920, must be a different work on the same subject if our author has the right date. Also, although Willy Schrödter credits Kilner with an M.D. he does not appear to have had one; however, as an M.R.C.P., he no doubt carried the courtesy title of "Dr." Tr.]; FEERHOW, Dr. Friedr., *Die menschliche Aura und ihre experimentelle Erforschung* [The Human Aura and Its Experimental Investigation] (Leipzig, 1914).

[280]BAGNALL, Oscar, *The Origin and Properties of the Human Aura* (London, 1937).

[281]TORMIN, Ludwig, *Magische Strahlen* [Magical Rays] (Düsseldorf, 1896).

[282]KNIESE, Julie, *. . . und es wird Licht* [. . . And There Is Light] (München-Solln, n.d.).

[283]HAUPT, pp. 33–34; MAACK, Dr. Ferd., *Das zweite Gehirn* [The Second Brain] (Hamburg, 1921), pp. 33, 34.

[284]MOUFANG, Dr. Wilh., *Magier, Mächte und Mysterien* [Magicians, Powers, and Mysteries] (Heidelberg, 1954), p. 271; SCHÄFER, *Das Fest der weißen Schleier* [The Festival of the White Veil].

laboratory of the University of Amsterdam in the presence of two assistants from the physical laboratory (of Prof. CLAY). The immigrant had to resign his apprenticeship as a photographer because every plate that passed through his hands was inexplicably traversed by black bands, "as if a mysterious effluvium had issued from the fingers that had held the plates." A search for radium salts under the nails proved negative.[285]

For the record, now we have come to mention the word *effluvium*, I first met the term *effluvia vitalia* [vital effluvia] in a book dated 1700 (GLOREZ, Andreas, *Eröffnetes Wunderbuch*, etc. [The Open Wonder-Book, etc.], Regensburg & Stadtamhof, p. 321.

MODERN SCIENCE AND THE AURA

The physician in charge at the Manfred-Curry Clinic in Dießen (Ammersee), Dr. Hans Adolf HÄNSCHE, gave a lecture in August 1958 to a large audience on the subject of "Medicine on the Move," in which he made significant remarks on earth rays and the electric field by which we are surrounded. "Research carried out quite a number of years ago has shown that earth is checkered with electric poles, and that there is a continuous energy exchange between Heaven and Earth. Many trees have been discovered that try to avoid negative radiation fields and therefore grow elsewhere, or, if they cannot do so, fail to thrive, or become completely deformed. If space has an electric field, it must follow that humans have one, too. The eternal dream has been to make this aura visible." Dr. HÄNSCHE exhibited images in which this human electric field could be seen: images of people with healthy constitutions, and images of people who were exhausted or ill. The electric field showed where the disease germ lay: "Today we can measure these things exactly," he said. "Great new possibilities would seem to flow from this."[286]

---

[285]RIJNBERK, p. 92.
[286]ANONYMOUS, "Die menschliche Aura sichtbar gemacht" [The Human Aura Made Visible] From *Müncher Merkur* August 6, 1958. (In the report in "The hidden world" some sentences are obviously out of sequence; I have transposed them [W. SCHR.]).

I shall mention one other source of some of these images: according to statements made by Dr. Manfred CURRY (1899–1953), HÄNSCHE managed to construct a field-strength meter the size of a typewriter case, with which he demonstrated without the shadow of a doubt that every man and woman is surrounded by an electric field, which varies in appearance according to whether one is dealing with a W(arm-front) type or a C(old-front) type. An electrode was pressed into the hand of the test subject, and the researcher surveyed the area immediately surrounding the test subject with an electric probe, measured the distances from the body at which given field strengths were obtained, compared them with the "norms," and drew an outline through the points found. In this way, a graphic representation of the individual field is made; and by studying the divergences from the "normal field lines" the physician is able to tell where the distribution of voltage in the machinery of the body is not as it should be. This enables an early diagnosis to be made.[287]

• • •

Several years ago the German press was humming with the following item of science news: "The human being is a radiator of infra-red rays. The evidence for this assertion stands in the center of the revolution in medical knowledge published in 1954 by a medical-physical research group of the Unterlahn district in Rheinland-Pfalz. The team, led by Dr. Ernst SCHWAMM (born in 1912), a medical practitioner in Obernhof/Lahn, and the physicist Johann Jost REEH (born in 1927), in Bad Ems, has succeeded in building a physical measuring apparatus for recording irregularities in the energy field of the body before the process becomes pathological."[288]

If, following HÄNSCHE, one were to draw the outline of these irregular changes in the energy field of the body, that is to say of the measured bulges and indentations in the infra-red radiation

---

[287]O. P., "Der elektr. gemessene Krebs" [Electrically Measured Cancer], *Neue Ill. Wschau.* (1959), 2 [January 11]: 1, 2, 23.
[288]SCHWAMM, Dr. Ernst, and REEH, J. J., "Die Ultrarotstrahlung des Menschen und seine Molekularspektroskopie" [Infra-Red Radiation in Humans and Its Molecular Spectroscopy], *Erfahr.hk.* (1954), 4: 151–157; SCHWAMM, Dr. Ernst, "Ultrarotstrahlung und Krebsgeschehen" [Infra-Red Radiation and the Course of Cancer], *Erfahr.hk.* (1954), 7: 313–317; SCHWAMM, "Die Ultrarot-strahlung und ihre medizinische Bedeutung" [Infra-Red Radiation and Its Medical Significance], *Erfahr.hk.* (1955), 11, 481–491, 12: 533–542.

enveloping the body, one would obtain aura contours as he did, and no doubt the auras would vary in type.

Two American scientists, Dr. W. S. HUXFORD and Dr. A. M. NETHERCOT of Northwestern University, are reported to have built a piece of apparatus in 1949 that converts the spoken word into infra-red rays, which can be picked up from as far away as 160 miles and turned back into sound by a suitable receiver.[289] Should it indeed turn out that telepathy depends on infra-red radiations, human beings would be incomparably better senders and receivers than all this fancy equipment. For one thing, human telepathy can reach anywhere on earth!

• • •

The well-known dowsing researcher and geophysicist, Dr. WÜST, is one of those who is said to have proved the existence of the human aura by exact measurements, such as are demanded and accepted by the scientific community. Each of us has an aura with its own special frequency. It has also been proved that this energy emission passes through glass practically undiminished. A small glass flask containing a liquid collects the radiation. Heat rays in the 10 μ range (= 0.01 mm) have been measured in the aura, and also electromagnetic radiations with wavelengths between a centimeter and a meter. The measuring equipment could hardly have been more simple: a paraffin concave mirror with a crystal (coherer-detector) at its focus collected the rays from the human fingertips and amplified them for measurement by the detector.

These experiments prove that during potentization [of homeopathic remedies by hand *Tr.*] the energies of the potentizer can be transmitted through the glass to the remedy.[290]

As regards "electromagnetic radiations with wavelengths between a centimeter and a meter": as long ago as 1930, Dr. M.

---

[289]"Unsichtbares Licht" als "Nachrichtenübertragungs-Apparat" ["Invisible light" as "a signalling apparatus"], *Neues Europa* (1949), 24 [Dec. 15]: 5.
[290]LINDER, Ferdinand, Das Problem der homöopathischen Hochpotenz [The Problem of Homeopathic High Potencies], *Naturhprax.* (1957), 7 [July]: 150; WÜST, Dr. Jos., "Physikalische und chemische Grundlagen der menschlichen Aura" [Physical and Chemical Bases of the Human Aura], *Neue Wiss.* (1954), 7: 193 f., 8–9 257; WÜST, "Probleme der Paraphysik [Problems of Paraphysics], *Neue Wiss.* (1953), 13: 377 f.; Anonymous, "Die starke Kraft der Verdünnungen" [The Strong Power of Dilution], *Zbl. Okk.* (1918), 2 [August]: 93.

MOINEAU was said to have "invented an apparatus with which he was able to measure the electromagnetic waves of the human body, which vary in strength and length from one person to another. He recorded lengths between 22 and 45 mm."[291]

As regards "coherer-detector," the use of this catchword confirms my belief that many see a "brain-coherer" in the solar plexus. WÜST thought it likely "that human beings have at their disposal in the vegetative nervous system a highly sensitive receiving apparatus that responds, not only to the weather and its effects, but also to telepathy."[292]

He found support in SCHLEICH: "Our solar plexus in the pit of the stomach is a wireless-telegraphy station, capable of receiving possible thought-telegrams."

• • •

Tests performed by Dr. S. W. TROMP (geological adviser to the UN) with an Einthoven electrocardiograph, have verified that each of us is surrounded by a physically measurable and clearly polar aura. "These tests are described in detail in *Psychical Physics* (1949; Elsevier Verlag). The various aspects of *Psychischen Physik* are studied in Holland by the Stiftung für psychische Physik [The Institution for Psychical Physics] (Office: Oostsingel 24, Delft), which was founded on July 18, 1950."[293]

• • •

The human reaction distance measurable with the dowsing rod was found by Dr. Wolff BLOSS general practitioner in Bietigheim (Württ.), without all this complicated apparatus, but by a slight sense of coldness in the palms of the hands as the reaction distance is traversed.[294]

---

[291]GARSCHAGEN, R., "Die Ausstrahlungen des menschlichen Körpers" [The Radiations of the Human Body], *Der Lebenskraftheiler* (1932), 6: 42. [After the *Journal du Magnétisme et du Psychisme expérimental*, 1932, November issue.]

[292]RINGGER, p. 45.

[293]TROMP, Dr. S. W., "Einzelne Aspekte der "Psychischen Physik" und die darüber in Holland im Gang befindlichen Untersuchungen" [Individual Apsects of "Psychical Physics" and Research Currently Being Performed in Holland]. *Neue Wiss.* (1954), 4 [April]: 119 f.

[294]BLOSS, Dr. W., "Ist der Reaktionsabstand mit den Händen erfühlbar?" [Is the Reaction Distance Perceptible by the Hands?], *Z. Radiästh.* (1936), 1936, 1–22, 23 f.; SCHRÖDTER, *Grenzwissenschaftliche Versuche* [Psychological Experiments], chapter on the Etheric Body.

In the 3–4 cm.-thick "cold mantle" observed in this way, I see an aura. This "palm of the hand phenomenon" associated here with a living (incarnate) person, has its counterpart in the temperature drop noticed in haunting by a discarnate (disembodied) spirit.

THE META-ORGANISM

The aura may be regarded as the projection of a subtle "inner body" beyond the confines of the physical body. Also, since it can extend further than usual, beyond the contours of the body, when the person is in a state of exaltation, the word "ecstasy," which comes from the Greek *ekstasis*, can also be derived from the Latin *ex-stare* (stand out). Now because the meta-organism is the starting-point of the aura, we need to take a look at it.

At all places and times, esotericism has alleged the existence of a "subtle body," from the *linga sharira* of the Indians to the "etheric body" of the Theosophists and the "formative forces body" of the Anthroposophists. The Islamic *Tarikaat* (secret doctrine) calls it *Djismi essiri*, and the retired teacher Hans HÄNIG speaks of the "electromagnetic substrate."[295] As a matter of fact, engineer Fritz GRUNEWALD (who died in 1925) experimentally located in his physical laboratory in Berlin-Charlottenburg "several magnetic centers, or poles, outside the body."[296] By those who are able to see them, the "chakras," (i.e., "wheels," also known as "lotuses") of ancient Indian occultism.[297] These are, "vortices in the

---

[295]HÄNIG, Hans, "Ausscheidung der Empfindung und Astralleib" [Evolution of Sensation and of the Astral Body], *Okk. Welt.* (n.d.), No. 176, p. 4.

[296]GRUNEWALD, Fritz, "Physikalisch-mediumistische Untersuchungen" [Physical and Mediumistic Researches], *Okk. Welt* (n.d.), No. 13–16, p. 54.

[297]AVALON, Arthur, (Sir John Woodroffe), *The Serpent Power* (London, 1919; Luzac. Madras 1918, 1950); BOHM, Werner, published in English as *Chakras, Yoga & Consciousness* (York Beach, ME: Samuel Weiser, 1991, 1998); LEADBEATER, Ch. W., *The Chakras* (Adyar, 1927); and *Die Chakras, Kraftzentren im menschlichen Ätherkörper* [The Chakras, Force Centers in the Human Etheric Body] (Düsseldorf, 1929); WACHSMUTH, Dr. Günth., *Bilder und Beiträge zur Mysterien- und Geistesgeschichte der Menschheit* [Pictures and Articles Illustrating the History of Human Thought and Human Mysteries] (Dresden, 1938), see chapter on "Metaphysical human organs in the East and the West."

etheric organism which, to those who perceive them, are experienced and seen as turning wheels which look something like flowers."[298] In general, seven are recognized, which mesh like gear wheels in the plexuses of the body's nervous system,[299] and with an equal number of endocrine glands.[300] What is more, the German hermetists—among whom were TRITHEMIUS, Basilius VALENTINUS, GICHTEL, and JUNG-STILLING—knew of them;[301] and the Rosicrucians referred to them as the "roses on the (back-) cross," which it is up to us to bring into bloom.

"May the roses *on* your cross bloom!" Surgeon colonel D. Rudolf MLAKER (born in 1889) of Vienna explored the state of development of the "vital centers."[302]

This "phantom body" has been made visible, photographed, and weighed. *"Phantom limb pains"* arise in it (SCHRÖDTER: opus sub 141).

MODERN SCIENCE AND THE "META-ORGANISM"

"We can also designate this subtle body as the "life field," as is done by the renowned scientist Dr. Gustav STRÖMBERG, director of the observatory of the Carnegie Institute on Mt. Wilson (1731 m) near Pasadena CA. This life field, which appears even in the embryo, reaches its fullest extent at maturity, then contracts at the time of death and quits the body for the non-physical world. According to Dr. STRÖMBERG, all our memories are contained in the "brain field," which must be regarded as part of the "life field." The structure and functions of living organisms and their organs are similarly determined and controlled by "organization fields." The brain field has a precisely bounded electrical structure,

[298]FRITSCHE, Dr. Herbert, *Der große Holunderbaum* [The Great Elder Tree] (Leipzig, 1939), p. 32.
[299]STRAUSS-SURYA, pp. 203–204; BIRVEN, p. 44.
[300]ROUSELLE, Erwin, *Mysterium der Wandlung* [The Mystery of Transformation] (Darmstadt, 1923), p. 54.
[301]v. SEBOTTENDORF (Leipzig), p. 43; (Freiburg i. B.), p. 49 f.
[302]MLAKER, Rudolf, *Geistiges Pendeln* [Spiritual Dowsing] (Villach, 1951).

which controls and maintains the structure and function of our brain. At death, the "memory field" withdraws from the physical brain and disappears from the physical world, although the form of its spiritual elements is preserved unchanged. Many of the electrical activities of this "life field" have been investigated by the Medical Faculty of Yale University in New Haven, CT. On the basis of recent knowledge, the erudite Prof. STRÖMBERG takes it as proved that human beings survive death because their memories survive.[303, 304]

• • •

The Hungarian scientist Prof. BRAVIAK even succeeded in fixing the force field or life field of a dying person as a blue light effect on an apparatus for half an hour beyond the point of death. And then, it would seem, with a sudden flaring and hissing, the apparatus was burned. The life field had finally left the corpse.[303] This research was carried out in April 1949 in a Budapest hospital in the presence of local scientists and top officials.[305]

• • •

The research of the Munich physician Dr. Dora ROHLFS (born in 1892) points in the same direction. She studied the "biological force field" . . . quite independently of other investigators. The biological force field can be implicated in mass just as the electromagnetic field of physics can, but it persists when the mass is removed. It is indestructible as long as its sender remains, and is like the life fields and the subtle body which continue to exist when our earthly covering decays.[303, 306]

---

[303]ROESERMUELLER, W. O., Unsere "Toten" leben [Our "Dead" Live] (Nuremberg, 1958), p. 23.
[304]STRÖMBERG, Dr. Gustav, The Soul of the Universe, The Searchers (Philadelphia: David Mc.Kac Company).
[303]See footnote above.
[305]LANDSBERG, Friedr., Die Seele wurde sichtbar [The Soul has Become Visible] (Sternzeit, 1949), 1 f.
[303]See footnote above.
[306]ROHLFS, Dr. Dora, Irrationales und rationales Erkennen [Irrational and Rational Perception] (Munich, 1950); FRANK, Dr. Otto, Die Bahn der Gestalt [The 'Gestalt' Way] (Flensburg, 1949).

AURIC LIGHT

When in the "Acts of the Apostles" (Ch. 5: 15) we read that ". . . they brought forth the sick into the streets, and laid them on beds and couches, that at least the *shadow* of PETER passing by might overshadow some of them." Then, according to RIJNBERK, "the shadow is just the symbolic representative of the vital, astral, fluid quintessence."[307] PAUL (died A.D. 62), who spoke of a subtle body (the *soma pneumatikon*),[308] also spoke of the differing glories[309] of our "wedding garment."[310] And if we see this in connection with the Lord's words that ". . . there is nothing covered that shall not be revealed; and hid, that shall not be known."[311] this could quite easily be interpreted as follows: one day, the moral level of each and all will become visible in the greater or less glory of the "spiritual body." Even here and now, the *Ilm el Miftach* already mentioned will make visible, by means of the systematically developed inner eye, the auric play of colors associated with evolution.[312] There is agreement in the relevant doctrines that dark colors indicate a low state of development, and light colors a high one. Chinese Yoga has an apt term for this: "the light of essential nature." In order to convey some idea of "auric sight," which many readers will surely find fascinating, here is a relevant experience of the well-known Munich parapsychologist Dr. Gerda WALTHER (born in 1897).

The account was published in advance as an extract from "a big book of memoirs now in preparation": It was one afternoon in 1922 "in the recess between the summer and winter semes-

---

[307]RIJNBERK, p. 197. A seriously ill person has hardly any aura. Peter Schlemihl does not cast a shadow.

[308]I Corinthians 15: 44.

[309]I Corinthians 15: 41.

[310]Matthew 22: 12. [A careful reading of the Bible passages quoted suggests that they are not referring to a subtle body possessed now in addition to the physical body and capable of surviving it, but of a spiritual body that will replace the present physical one on the day of resurrection. The two concepts are different. Again, the wedding garments were bestowed on the guests, they were not something they had had all along—as would have been the case if they were analagous to the aura. *Tr.*].

[311]Matthew 10: 26.

[312]v. SEBOTTENDORF, (Leipzig edition), p. 41; (Freiburg i. B. edition), p. 47.

ters," when our informant, who was then staying in Darmstadt, set out at an agreed time to keep an appointment. "Now, as I was walking down Nieder-Ramstädter Street I felt, on coming to a sharp bend, as if I had run into something that could be compared to a strong psychic or spiritual magnetic current. What could it be? On the left-hand side it was weaker. It fell across the street like a deep shadow, and became stronger and stronger on the right. There stood, half turned away, the figure of a man in front of a shop window. He was only of medium build, yet I noticed with astonishment how, apart from the "magnetic force field," he was surrounded by a brilliantly clear golden-white aura, which gave him twice as big an effect on his surroundings as anyone else. So who was he? GEORGE of course—Stefan George!

Fairly slowly I went on my way, as if suffused with this glittering radiance . . . , what surprised me was that it did not grow weaker the further I got from the shop window."[313]

AURIC DIAGNOSIS

However, the color of Od shows not only the moral character of its carrier, but also his or her state of health:

> People in perfect physical and mental health appear to trance subjects in a predominantly blue or blue-green Od-light; those who are unwell or immoral in a predominantly brown or red Od-light. So it would seem that the Od is closely connected with health and disease. REICHENBACH'S sensitives repeatedly predicted coming diseases several days in advance, simply on the basis of the change they observed in his Od-light, and the prediction invariably came true. Inflamed areas and organs had a bright red glow, enabling the sensitives to indicate to him the exact site of the disease.[314]

---

[313]WALTHER, Dr. Gerda, "Eine nicht alltäglich Begegnung mit dem Dichter Stefan George" [An Unusual Encounter with Poet Stefan George], *Neue Wiss.* (1958), 9 [Nov./Dec.].
[314]RIEDLIN, p. 179.

The Spanish physician, Dr. Francisco DI BORJA DE SAN ROMAN employs "Aura-diagnosis." During healing magnetic treatment, he looks for a correction of the diseased aura, which can be detected by someone who is naturally gifted in the use of the pendulum, the so-called "rotating divining rod."[315]

German doctors have been writing books for several decades now on the use of the pendulum and the dowsing rod in diagnosis.[316]

AURIC THERAPY

Dr. WALTHER expressed astonishment that the bright radiance of Stefan GEORGE did not become weaker as she moved further away from him. It is obvious that with greater or less illuminating power, the range of the aura is greater or less. Therefore primitive medicine has graded the limits of "auric protection."

"The notion that the human body radiates individual emanations, possibly forms the starting point for the rules imposed on the *Brahmans* of Malabar concerning separation from so-called "unclean" persons belonging to other castes. For example: a *Sudra* defiles a Brahmin if he approaches him by less than 3 to 6 paces; a *Mezillah* (Moslem of Malabar) from 6 through 12 paces; a menstruating woman at 12 paces; a woman who has only recently given birth, at 18 paces. Thus the unconscious perception of the body's emanations possibly forms the esoteric basis of a conception of cleanness that one encounters both in the Far East and the Near East."[317]

On the evening of October 7, 1827, GOETHE was sitting in the "Zum Bären" hostelry with his [friend and secretary] ECKERMANN, and said to the latter: "We all have something in the way of electrical and magnetic forces in us and, like the magnet itself, we possess a power of attraction and repulsion in accor-

---

[315]E. B. "Ist Ihre Aura krank?" [Is Your Aura Diseased?], *Neues Europa* (1956), 21.

[316]CLASEN, Dr. Ernst, *Die Pendeldiagnose* [Pendular Diagnosis] (Leipzig, 1929); VOLL, Dr. A., *Wünschelrute und siderisches Pendel* [Dowsing Rod and Pendulum] (Leipzig, 1910); WEISS, Dr. Karl Erhard, *Der siderische Pendel im Reiche des Feinstofflichen* [The Sidereal Pendulum in the Realm of Fine Matter].

[317]RIJNBERK, p. 96.

dance with whether we come in contact with something like or unlike."*

The distinguished private scholar Surya came to the same conclusion in 1907, and used the same example. Within a short time his familiarity with Dr. Nicolson produced in him a new spiritual life. *It was as if the mere presence of the latter was sufficient to arouse elevated thoughts in him and feelings which, until then, had only lain slumbering.*

The academic learning of today wishes to know nothing of this sort of powerful influence exerted by a highly developed person on others! And yet nature teaches us that even a so-called inanimate body, such as a piece of steel, can possess hidden powers and properties, which we are unable to perceive with our coarse senses even though they can produce perfectly clear and lasting effects in other bodies. Thus, the mere "presence" of a powerful steel magnet is enough to deflect all the magnet needles in its proximity and even to reverse their polarity in some circumstances?[318]

The American Japanese Hiro Hasegawa, instructor in Jujitsu in the police academies in the state of California and later in Chicago, devoted an entire chapter of his textbook[319] to the "psychology of Jujitsu." He writes:

You must be clear about one thing in every struggle in which you are engaged. You do not act on your opponent by your physical movements alone—not by your grips, thrusts, and throws alone. More importantly, an immediate impact is made by your whole being, or body-soul unit. . . . The secret of psychic influence on the opponent will be understood by those who study the old Eastern philosophies. They really comprehend how the radiations act. According to these doctrines, each of us is surrounded by a personal radiation field, through which we touch our environment. Its essence, which consists of mind and body, of thoughts and actions, acts through space like a magnet. If the thoughts are strong and confident, they have a coercive ef-

---

*I have kept Goethe's word order: "attraction . . . repulsion" and "like . . . unlike." In magnetism, of course, it is unlike poles that attract and like poles that repel.

[318]Surya, *Rosenkreuzer* [The Rosicrucians], p. 73.

[319]Hasegawa, Hiro, *Jiu-Jitsu-Judo. Die Kunst der Selbstverteidigung* [Jujitsu or Judo. The Art of Self-Defense], (German translation by Hch. Krafft), (Lindau, n.d.), pp. 70–71.

*fect. Now strength, confidence, and composure are part of the
nature of the Jujitsu fighter.*

The *auric heterodyne*—to borrow a striking word from radio technology—can bring about a fluid discharge from the agent, and
thus a reinforcement of the "counterpart," as in the law of com-
municating vessels. This would be the purely Odic activity. But
one may assume that it is equally possible to produce a synchronized commutation. And then there is something more; namely
the "impartation of a cross section of the other person's nature,"
or a "participation" (Latin: *communio*) in the "light of essential
nature." Of course, the two effects can be produced simultane-
ously (collectively).

In my opinion, just such a "compound effect" seems to have
occurred in the following case, in which the mental attitude of
the person generating the impulse need not concern us: "(This)
true story is about something that happened in a Berlin suburb.
A relatively young man had suffered a stroke, being completely
paralyzed, and apparently in a coma. The doctor declared that
death was inevitable and would supervene within a few hours.
The man's family was reduced to a state of absolute despair. His
wife and daughter implored the doctor to do something. He told
them that that was impossible. 'There is nothing more to be
done,' he said; which only made them more frantic. Then he
added, 'Although I myself can do nothing, someone I will fetch
for you may do some good—perhaps.'

"The doctor hurried to see a man who was a Christian Scientist and whose mysterious therapeutic success had come to his
ears. Only the man's 14-year-old daughter was at home, and the
doctor told her why he had come. 'Take me to the sick man,' offered the girl, 'I will heal him!' Reluctantly the doctor agreed, and
not long afterward the child entered the room in which the sick
man was lying immobile with the death rattle in his throat.

"She sat on the edge of the bed, without saying a word and
without stirring. After half an hour he sat up and said: 'Give me
something to eat!' An hour later he left his bed and was perfectly
well.

"'What did you do to the sick man?' the doctor asked the
girl. She replied, 'I realized that the man had forgotten that God

is his life, *and I brought this back to his consciousness.'* The news was picked up by a reporter . . . the authenticity of the case was confirmed to him by the doctor and by several other persons."[320]

The source from which I have taken the above report is opposed to Christian Science and I myself regard it as neither "Christian" nor "science." What is more, it is not a *theurgic* mode of therapy or "faith-healing," but a monoideistic "thought-healing"! But this plays no part in the occasional certified successes it has notched up: it is immaterial what the thoughts are to which the encourager or the patient elevate their minds. The father of the youthful healer possibly had a natural gift, but plucked up the courage to work as a healer only after joining the movement founded in the USA by Mary BAKER-EDDY (1821–1910) in 1866. The healing gift may then have been inherited by his daughter, who—having been encouraged by the healing sect—found the necessary confidence in the gift at an earlier age than her parent did.

OBJECTS IMPREGNATED WITH THE AURA

The emotional charge of the aura impregnates, for example, the paper on which we write a letter. It adheres to the paper for a certain time and enters the recipient when the letter is held in the hands.[321] The recipient may catch the mood in which the letter was written, even though there are no clues in the actual words. The strength of the transfer depends on the degree of excitement (and innervation) of the sender, on the degree of sensibility of the recipient, and on the closeness of the contact between them. If the writers are the personification of good will, as SURYA was, and if, in addition, they were animated by a keen desire to help, the possibility of their favorably influencing physical sufferers through letters impregnated with their aura should not be dismissed out of hand. If complete syntonizing (consonance) occurs, the assimi-

---

[320]FOURNIER, Christine, *Das Reich der Gottes-Hysterie.* ["Christian Science" The Kingdom of Divine Hysteria], Prophets in the German crisis: The Miraculous or the Bewitched, The Rudolf OLDEN collection (Berlin, 1932), p. 161 f.

[321]MOUFANG, p. 10; after GREBER, Rev. Johannes, *Der Verkehr mit der Geisterwelt etc.* [Intercourse with the Spirit World] (New York, 1937).

lated impulse may be enough to reactivate the repressed ent-elechy (the "Archaeus" of PARACELSUS). To sum up, it is the *vis med-icatrix naturae* of the sick person that effects the cure. The healer "only" contributes the missing, and possibly quite small, differ-ence ("restoration subsidy") that is necessary to bring the ent-elechial "watering can" back to the state in which it can "water the vegetation of the body." So far we have been considering the purely Odic aspect. But some mental block, which has resisted the natural recuperative powers, can be removed by odically-fixed, emotionally-toned thoughts ("disinhibition"). This would not ac-tually be due to Od,[322] but would be a telepathic-auric action on the psyche! Perhaps such impulses are the primary ones more often than one might think. Thus a lady doctor practicing in Mu-nich wrote the following to me on February 4, 1959:

> *In one case, where I had given the patient up, but did inject directly into his heart without his regaining consciousness during the space of time I remained in attendance, I myself do* not *believe that it was exclusively the injection that revived him, but that a psychic impulse was actively received during the crisis. We doctors have evidence that it is* only *the medi-cines that work in such cases, and yet to prove it . . .*

In discussing *Boltzianism* we have already touched on the fact that clothes can be impregnated with Od, but have dealt only with the therapeutic side of the subject. There is, however, an-other side. Let Cornelius AGRIPPA point it out to us: "They say that a woman who puts on the gown or shift of a whore becomes im-pudent, bold, shameless, and impure.[323] Like me, Gustav JAEGER, who has given a lot of thought to clothing ("Wool-regime Jaeger") and to the closely connected subject of Od[324] would not

---

[322]KRAMER, Phil. W., *Der Heilmagnetismus* [Animal Magnetism], (Leipzig, 1907), A disserta-tion by Lud. Tormin), p. 109.

[323]AGRIPPA, vol. I, p. 107.

[324]JAEGER, Gustav, *Selbstarznei und Heilmagnetismus* [Self-Treatment and Animal Magnet-ism] (Stuttgart, 1908); KRÖNER, Dr. Walter, *Die Metabiologie Gustav Jaegers: Ketzermedizin gestern—Neuralmedizin heute* [The Metabiology of Gustav Jaeger: Yesterday's Quackery—Today's Neuraltherapeutics] (Ulm/Donau: Karl F. Haug Verlag, 1955).

dismiss this piece of folk-wisdom with a superior smile. Thus, for example, he has stated that it is a sign of very great affection if one person can put on another person's bathing suit. Be that as it may; an unused piece of clothing lacks that certain *je ne sais quoi* possessed by one that is worn!

This brings me to the subject of the warm chair seat, which is deeply disliked by nearly all of us if it has just been vacated by a stranger. If a seat were infected with a neutral Od, it could not be found unpleasant by the next occupant. At all events, in my own experience it hardly bothers me if I sit on a seat that has just been used by a member of my own family. There is an odic affinity between us, which is certainly the reason why we would rather accept the chair of a relative we get on with than that of someone we do not take to. Organic animal heat is quite different from inorganic physically produced heat. On this subject no less a person than the physician in ordinary to the king of Saxony, Dr. Carl Gustav CARUS (1789–1869) voiced the following opinion:

> *Even the casual observer will notice that, for example, the warmth of a healthy soft human hand has a quite different effect on us from the same degree of heat (as measured by a thermometer) in a piece of iron or wood; and that the breath of someone we love affects us differently from a flow of damp air at the same temperature issuing from a steam-heater.*[325]

That all heat is not the same heat is also demonstrated by the incubation heat of birds. The ornithologist and forester Johann Matthäus BECHSTEIN (1757–1822) "put eggs from black pigeons under a red jacobin and the young pigeons were spotted with red and closely resembled their foster-mother, which would never happen in the ordinary way."[326] What is more: "The incubation heat of the hen is (actually) slightly luminous, as anyone can observe in the dry season."[327]

---

[325]CARUS, p. 105.

[326]PASSAVANT, Dr. Joh. Carl, *Untersuchungen über den Lebensmagnetismus und das Hellsehen* [Researches into Biomagnetism and Clairvoyance] (Frankfurt/Main, 1837).

[327]SCHWAEBLÉ, René, *Alchimie simplifié* (Paris: Librairie du Magnétisme, n.d.), p. 34.

ANOTHER LOOK AT AMULETS

As I have already shown, cloth and paper are easily charged with Od. Now many amulets are kept in a cloth receptacle (the "medicine bag" of the Indians!), or may consist of paper (parchment, "virgin parchment"), on which some protective formula or curse (spell) is written or some magic sigil is drawn.

The effect of the amulet can be explained by the presence of Od, but it is preferable to think of it in terms of the aura: the object is emotionally charged by the amulet-maker for a considerable time until it becomes an amulet. As we are informed by STRINDBERG, who had studied medicine, an accumulator of psychic power is "not any more remarkable than an electric torch, which gives light on two conditions: that it has a live battery and that the button is pressed. Amulets, too, have conditions and do not work in all circumstances." An amulet "can impart strength to those who possess the necessary receiving apparatus—'faith'."[328]

DAVID-NEEL seconds the great Swede: "(In Tibet) one can charge an object with these (thought-waves) as one charges an electric accumulator, and can then draw on the stored energy for any given purpose, such as to increase the vitality of the person touched by the object, or to make him intrepid, and so on."[329]

The secret doctrine of Ancient India spoke of such thought waves aimed at an object for the purpose of charging it, as *Pitta currents*: we ourselves follow VON REICHENBACH in calling them "psychic dynamides."

HUMAN RADIATION REVEALS HUMAN NATURE

So states Prof. Eugen MATTHIAS (born in 1882) of Zürich, and he has demonstrated it, so he tells us, with the help of a special apparatus. And he adds, "An unbroken chain of evidence leads to

---

[328] STRINDERG, August, *Ein Blaubuch* [A Blue Book] (Munich, 1920), chapter on "accumulators".

[329] DAVID-NEEL, p. 272.

the conclusion that the penetrating power of human radiations can impinge on such items as the written page, photographs, *objets d'art*, and even on very old historic documents, and can return from these things unaltered as if they were coming from the person who emitted them."[330]

I myself have put it this way: "The emanations of the being and doing (of a person) bury themselves in the assimilating material (paper, linen, stone, etc.), and can re-emerge in their original form and magnitude. MATTHIAS uses the term *penetration* for this phenomenon which, in my opinion, seems to explain the fact of *psychometry* and *talismans*."[331] The penetration detected by a piece of apparatus working automatically would provide objective proof of the possibility of mentally charging objects (as has been maintained by believers in amulets in every time and place), and would provide it in a way that the pendulum (whether fixed or not) could never do, since the latter is brought in contact with the human hand.

To begin with, the results of the Swiss research-worker have to be verified, and he needs to give a complete and accurate description of his apparatus in a subsequent volume. It is quite understandable that he will not do so while his patent application is being processed.

Should his, and his publishers' statements turn out to be true, his research method is—to put it in a nutshell—"comprehensive." Certainly if, for example, as he has intimated to other scientists, it has been possible since December 18, 1954 "to determine the exact blood pressure, both maximum and minimum, and also the amplitude and the biggest pulsation in the blood pressure, from a piece of writing"! Just now I have received from his publishers the news that this researcher, who was born in Alstätten bei Zürich in 1882, died in Zürich in April 1958. "It is still not known if his second book on radiations will be published. And nothing definite can be said at present about the continua-

---

[330]MATTHIAS, Prof. Eugen, *Die Strahlen des Menschen künden sein Wesen* [Human Radiations Reveal Human Nature] (Zürich, 1955). Note by Europa Verlag AG on the dust-jacket.
[331]SCHRÖDTER, Willy, "Die Strahlen des Menschen künden sein Wesen" [Human Radiations Reveal Human Nature], *Mensch und Schicksal* (1956), 22 [February 1]: 7 f.

tion of his scientific work." Graduated engineer Artur FLASSER (born in 1886) held the following view, which I have made my own: "Like the pendulum, the apparatus of MATTHIAS is exposed to subjective influences. This is evidenced both by the testing of objects which emit no rays and are not surrounded by fields—for example a printed poem of GOETHE's—and also by misjudgments concerning some objects. It is possible that the dowser is included in the circuit, and that the apparatus reproduces the thought of the dowser—here VON MATTHIAS. Nevertheless the equipment is a definite advance, and has to be regarded as a discovery in the area of pendulum diagnosis. The enlistment of pH measurement is a very good idea."

THE HUMAN ATMOSPHERE

The words "aura" and "atmosphere" are quite often synonymous in both German and English; but like most synonyms, they do have different shades of meaning. Individual auras vary not only in luminosity, but also in the extent to which they stream out beyond the contours of the body (Latin: *ex-stare*). This extent probably increases in states of ecstasy or exaltation. At all events, *the direct action and maximum effect of the aura occur in proximity to the body* ("Walking in the aura of the anointed").

However, just as a radiator heats the air, and using the air as a carrier goes on to heat the floor, walls, and ceiling of a room, so the auric "radiator," also using the air as a medium, impregnates the room to its periphery, clings to the walls and adheres to the furniture. The primary reference of the word "atmosphere" is to the gaseous envelopes of the planets, but first and foremost to the one belonging to Earth. This is the air that surrounds us, but there is a secondary reference to the spiritual environment in which we live, whether created by ourselves or by others. And others or we ourselves react to it as the case may be. The fact that the word "air" is not used in this sense, but another word (i.e., "atmosphere") seems to show, in my opinion, that the air in a room occupied by humans is not regarded as completely neutral! *Thus the atmosphere is the peripheral effect of the aura.*

PERIPHERAL EFFECTS ON OTHER HUMAN BEINGS

The following quotations bear out what has just been said above:

CORNELIUS AGRIPPA (1510)

"Therefore the philosophers warn against associating with evil-minded and unfortunate people, because their souls are filled with harmful radiations which will *infect your surroundings in an unhealthy way*. On the contrary, one should seek the company of good and fortunate people, for these can help us greatly *by being near to us*" [I, 316].

PARACELSUS (CA. 1530)

"A spiritual force resides in true self-awareness and can be transferred from the physician to the patient, provided the latter possesses it. With its help, *the mere presence of the doctor* does the patient more good than any amount of medicine. For the etheric vibrations penetrate the human ether and are then able to convert the sick person's inharmonic vibrations into harmonic ones."

H. W. DRESSER (1902)

The spiritual healer "accordingly tries to be open and free in spirit" [13]. "If one has become open and free in this way, one can then turn and *surround* the sufferer in the same calm but strong and invigorating spirit *with an atmosphere that is so powerful* that no inharmonic mental or physical state can withstand it for long" [14].

MAGNETIZER LUDWIG TORMIN (1907)

"Albrecht VON HALLER and later HUMBOLDT and REIL have put forward the theory that there is a *mental atmosphere* surrounding each organism which is perceptible by any foreign organism. The more intense this influence is, the more intimate is the blending of the odic exhalations. But because this odic exhalation issues more or less from the whole body, *the mere presence of a healthy person can often be beneficial to one who is ill.*"[332]

JULES LERMINA (DIED 1915)

"Disease is not purely physical, it is equally psychic; indeed, we might go so far as to say that it is especially psychic. Hate and anger are no less poisons than arsenic and strychnine—they are stronger, too. The ill-will of the evil person injures others. *He poisons with his malice the atmosphere of those he hates.*"[333]

DR. FRIEDRICH MARKUS HUEBNER (1934)

"As a matter of fact, one can be poisoned not only by unwholesome food, gases, and microbes, but also by unwholesome people. *What takes up the poison first of all is our invisible atmosphere*, which, so to speak, becomes negatively charged by contact with harmful radiations. This then has dangerous repercussions on mind and body. Only so can we explain the more powerful reactions we can display at the sight of someone with a malignant aura: sudden giddiness, stomach cramps, perspiration, and fits of crazy laughter or wild crying. Our organism is hard put to throw off an intoxication that menaces it or already seems to be active."[334]

DR. FRANZ VÖLGYESI (1948)

"The emanation from the weak soul is spare and weak. The radiating magnetic forces of the strong soul, on the other hand, are capable of shaking the world—and they do shake it."[335]

EGON M. HEIN (1951)

"Once on the occasion of a visit in 1932 to a lady suffering from chronic bronchitis, the author observed that all her unpleasant symptoms disappeared, *in a flash* (to use but one example) *as soon*

[332]KRAMER, pp. 106–107; BUTTENSTEDT, p. 120.
[333]LERMINA, Jules, *Die Geheimlehre. Praktische Magie* [Occultism: Practical Magic] (Leipzig, n.d.), p. 135.
[334]HUEBNER, p. 38.
[335]VÖLGYESI, *Seele* (Souls), p. 25 f.

as he entered her room."[336] The entrance of a fundamentally good person, full of inner piety, into a sick-room, often purifies *the atmosphere through their mere presence.*[337] Rather melodramatically, HEIN heads the tenth section of his booklet: "Altruism as the most important factor in every healing."

MUHAMMAD SUBUH (BORN IN 1901)

In 1958, wider circles in West Germany first heard tell of the "Subud" movement founded by "Pak" (little father) Subuh, which has its offices at Heimstätten-Allee 16, Planegg bei Munich. Twice a week 10 to 15 adherents come together for a so-called *latihan* and make themselves, so to speak, "inwardly empty." "*Upon which they suddenly feel a wonderful elevating force in themselves, which seems to be imparted to them by Pak Subuh and his wife.*"[338]

When the English inaugurator of "Subud"—J. G. BENNETT— met Muhammad SUBUH at Croydon airport in London on May 22, 1957, he "was impressed by two things: one was the ordinariness of his appearance, and the other was the sense of complete calm and detachment *which not only came from him but entered into me also as soon as I saw him.*"[339]

The former government officer from Middle Java declares that all he does is to release the forces in people. The origin of these forces is in the individual himself or herself, for the soul is responsive to the divine omnipotence—SUBUH could also say with "Master Axel" in the "Axel" of Philippe-Auguste Mathias Count DE VILLIERS DE L'ISLE ADAM (1840–1889) "I do not teach, I awaken!"

The awakening (or "opening" as it is called) that precedes the latihan, is certainly not always pleasant. Much depends on the moral level. Many are literally brought to the ground by the knowledge of their current evolutionary state, as I have learned from an English participant. The silent influence of one person on

---

[336]HEIN, Egon M., *Atomare Heilkräfte. Entdeckungen und Erkenntnisse auf dem Gebiet des Heilmagnetismus* [Atomic Healing Forces: Discoveries and Realizations in the Field of Animal Magnetism] (Vienna, 1951), p. 59.

[337]HEIN, p. 9.

[338]"Magier enthüllt sein geheimnis" [Magician Discloses his Secret], *Heim u. Welt* (1958), 10 [March 7]: 1, 12.

[339]BENNETT, J.G., *Concerning Subud* (New York: University Books, 1959), p. 50.

another in Subud is reminiscent of the *Heart*—or *Abu-Bekr-Zikr* of the *Nakshi-Bendi dervishes*.[340]

PERIPHERAL EFFECTS ON "DEAD" OBJECTS

Naturally, the peripheral effect on "dead" objects cannot be perceived directly, but only by its reflex action on humans.[341] Eira HELLBERG (Stockholm) kept a record of many relevant experiences as she went around the globe in search of mysteries. First of all, she paints the general picture for us:

> *Have you never had the feeling, when looking for a new (she means "another" [W. SCHR.]) apartment, that there is something unpleasant in the walls? Have you ever noticed in a hotel room an* atmosphere *that has nothing to do with the air and cleanliness? An atmosphere that exhales something distinctly human? Has there ever crept over you, when you are waiting in a room in a strange house, a room where everything is apparently congenial—the wallpaper, the furniture, the carpets, the colors, and the tasteful arrangement of everything—an uncomfortable sense of oppression? The hosts come in, and are agreeable, kindly, and friendly, but your uneasy feeling will not go away.[342] If our amiable hosts in their comfortable room cannot overcome our uneasiness, the reason is that the room and the objects in it are* saturated *with the mental activity of the occupants, their will- and thought-waves, which are beamed back on any receptive individual who comes within range of them.[343]*

I have already shown how a room can be charged with energy in the example of the consultation room of a mesmerist. A further example is given by BENNETT in his description of the latihan held

---

[340]VETT, Carl, *Seltsame Erlebnisse in einem Derschkloster* [Strange Experiences in a Dervish Monastery] (Straßburg, 1931), p. 103; and *Dervish Diary* (Los Angeles, 1953).

[341]AGRIPPA, Book. I, chapter 6.

[342]HELLBERG, p. 136.

[343]HELLBERG, p. 137.

on May 10, 1957 in the Lodge at Coombe Springs (England) for the Hungarian film star Eva BARTOK (born in 1929):

> *The little bedroom was charged with energy that annihilated all personal feeling and produced a state of consciousness in which all seemed to be sharing in one and the same experience as the sick woman.*[344]

This concentrated energy resulted in a steady improvement in Eva BARTOK's condition from the next morning onward, so that she did not need the scheduled operation. And, in October, she was successfully delivered of a healthy baby. "One has a sense of constriction in a room, and it turns out that the previous lodger had made away with himself. Thus something of his intense despair has been left behind in the room."[345] This can affect subsequent tenants. The following story has become a classic:

> *A sentry committed suicide in his sentry-box; He was immediately replaced by another, who also took his own life. The third and fourth soldiers did the same. NAPOLEON I ordered the sentry-box to be burned and that brought this uncanny suicide epidemic to an end.*[346]

The scene of the events was Boulogne-sur-Mer (Eberh. BUCHNER).

Surely our explanation on the basis of "atmospheres" is more straightforward than the suggestion that the spirits of the suicides were trying to make the relieving guards do away with themselves?

The chairman of a local authority once told me that a certain room in his office building seemed to have a peculiar effect on his staff. Sexual misbehavior was a constant problem there. He arranged for the builders to make some structural alterations and sex flew out of the window! "Many thoughts seem to be circling round in the air. Which is why it happens that the new lodger—

---

[344]BENNETT, p. 68.

[345]SCHRÖDTER, Willy, *Ausflug ins Wundersame* [An Excursion into the Supernatural] (Freiburg i.B., 1939), p. 53.

[346]FRICHET, p. 152.

provided he or she has the necessary sensitivity—assumes the inclinations, or even the characteristics, of a completely unknown predecessor, even while feeling that they are not being altogether true to themselves. Take for example the immigrant lady who had never cared for music, but suddenly felt an urge to perform music. It turned out that the lady who had previously occupied her room had hammered away on the piano day and night. Incidentally, the instrument was no longer there!"[347]

SÉDIR, who saw through to the underlying nature of things, believed that: "Human beings exercise a real influence on the objects in their environment. A chair that has been flung across the room in a rage stores anger inside it; the things used by a niggardly housewife make subsequent owners stingy."[348]

The "apostle of the miraculous" STERNEDER tells of an old patrician Viennese family who suffered inexplicable ill-health for two years. A clairvoyant friend identified an oil-painting in the sitting-room as a "hate-radiator." It had been purchased two years earlier, and after it was burned, the family members were revitalized. "For some reason, this picture was painted by the artist in a spirit of great hatred" said their "Janus-faced" friend.[349]

SCHLEICH informs us that when he visited his friend STRINDBERG in Stockholm: "All the furniture and other objects with which he surrounded himself seemed to be new, because he was determined not to have any old thoughts or feelings hanging about him." To be sure, one can interpret this as meaning that the old furniture and objects would have been constant reminders of the past: but the great Swede's knowledge of the hidden springs of everything allows us to interpret him along the lines laid down above.

MEYRINK portrayed in masterly fashion the influence exerted on the living by the dead through the things that had meant a lot to them and had been charged with their wishes.[350]

---

[347]SCHRÖDTER, *Ausflug* [An Excursion], p. 53.

[348]SÉDIR, Paul, *Les Forces mystiques et la Conduite de la Vie* [Mystical Forces and the Conduct of Life] (Bihorel-lez-Rouen (S. I.), 1923), p. 172 f.

[349]STERNEDER, Hans, *Frühling im Dorf* [Spring in the Village] (Leipzig, 1929), 249 f. SCHRÖDTER, Willy, "Gespensternde Bilder" [Spectral Pictures], *Natur u. Kultur* (1956), 1 [January]: 21.

[350]MEYRINK, Gust., *Der weiße Dominikaner* [The White Dominican] (Munich/Leipzig/Berlin/Vienna, 1921), pp. 267–272.

Eira HELLBERG describes a case in which a room that did not disturb the humans who used it, had a sinister effect on animals. He recalled that when he was a boy: "We never managed to get one dog into a certain corner (of the big parlor). We tugged her collar, tempted her with tidbits, begged or ordered her—but all in vain: she would press herself against the floor, whimpering with fear and displaying every sign of aversion. When we left the spot she leapt around us with delight.

"Our inquiries revealed that some years earlier the house had been occupied by a learned man and that he had set up a laboratory in this room. In the corner in question stood the bench and cage that he used for vivisection and for keeping the animals whose limbs he had paralyzed with *curare*. And that was the spook. It was not animal ghosts prowling around whining! But everything the creatures had suffered there was discharged and was absorbed by the walls, the floor, and the ceiling, where it was perceptible by animals of the same species.

"For as nerves can receive energy of enormous potential, and can also emit it by willed thought, should it not be possible for the organism's radiated energy either to enter into a chemical reaction with the surrounding objects or to be left partially unchanged?"[351]

As far as the "energy of enormous potential emitted by nerves" is concerned, here is an example from the animal world, which the well-known mesmerist, Prof. Carl Alexander Ferdinand KLUGE (1782–1844) thought worth mentioning: "COTUGNO wanted, for instance, to dissect a small house mouse while it was still alive, and caught hold of it by the skin of its back with two fingers and held it aloft. But, when the tail of the mouse touched his hand, he felt a heavy blow and a cramp that spread up his arm and shoulders to his head, leaving behind a painful sensation which lasted for a quarter of an hour."[352]

And now the equivalent from the human world: on October 18, 1818 in the Munich hospital, the 24-year-old country-girl A. S. gave an electric shock from a distance (!) to Mr B., who was talking to her when she was in an extremely excitable state (passing

---

[351]HELLBERG, pp. 137–138.
[352]KLUGE: pp. 241–242; §204.

through a bad crisis). She then shouted with horrible laughter: "Did you feel that? If only I had been able to get closer to you, you would have felt more."[353]

Having spoken of the room, HELLBERG goes on to speak of the house and its atmosphere: "There are some old houses in which new occupants feel unhappy and depressed without being able to say why; only when they no longer have to live in them do they regain their zest for life. Neither arsenic in the wallpaper nor rats under the floorboards can serve as an explanation for this, but only the lingering on of all that has happened there in the past."[354]

We might add that there is not in a new building the "certain something" that—doubtless perceptible by all of us—pleases us in a lived-in (one might almost say "cosy") house. (Besides, occupied houses last longer than unoccupied ones!) A Bible passage that is often overlooked hints at the "vitalizing" of a building.[355] "And when ye (the disciples) come into a house, salute it! And if the house be worthy, let your peace come upon them (the people living in the house): but if *it* be not worthy, let your peace return to you."

The peace greeting or benediction (in Hebrew: *Berachah*) is seen here as something material (ARAM). Just as it leaves an unworthy house and returns to the apostles, so a hundred years ago a Moslem still asked for his blessing back if he had bestowed it on an "infidel" by mistake.[356] "The reality of *mental atmospheres* becomes obvious even to a hard-boiled person, when he dwells on the vivid contrast between ballroom and courtroom, house of God and slaughterhouse, cemetery and brothel."[357]

The reality of a mental atmosphere throws light on an experience which is not grounded on real estate. We refer to the fact

---

[353]"Blätter für höher Wahrheit" [Papers for the Promotion of Higher Truth], Edited by Joh. Friedr. von Meyer: Selection I. XIII (Frankfurt/M: Archiv f. d. Thier, 1818), 290, 314; *Magnetismus* [Mesmerism], Besprechung von Nees von Esenbeck (Leipzig, 1817 f.), vol. V, 155–161; SCHRÖDTER, Willy, "Vom. Elektr. Menschen [Electric People], in *Mensch u. Schicksal* (1952), No. 19, of December 15, 8–13.
[354]HELLBERG, p. 138.
[355]Matthew 10: 12–13 [The Greek word for "house" in this passage also means "household." (See any good Greek lexicon). Therefore it is more likely that Jesus was telling His disciples to "salute the household" rather than the building itself. *Tr. note.*]
[356]RIJNBERK, p. 99.
[357]SCHRÖDTER, *Ausflug* [Excursion], p. 35.

that it is not all the same whether we listen to a symphony concert on the radio at second hand, or are present at the concert hall during the performance. And, clearly, listening to the broadcast of a carnival procession does not fully capture for us the infectious enthusiasm of the crowd.

The "naturally sighted" human being of prehistoric times possessed magical abilities and supersenses, remnants of which are still retained by nomadic tribes. But even these remnants have been lost by modern, almost completely extravert, civilized people. Our biologically and constitutionally given psychomagic has been increasingly replaced by the crutches of technomagic.[358] "Long-distance communications, long-distance conversations, and long-distance viewing are now no longer psychic, but are provided by telephone, telegraph, radio, and fax."[359] When Paul Joseph GOEBBELS (1897–1945) had to work through the night in the Ministry of Propaganda, he would call Lyda BAAROVA in her Grunewald villa and ask her to stay on the phone while he carried on working so that *at least she was with him in this way.*[360] But this is exactly where the powerlessness of technomagic lies: "One cannot send oneself and cannot cause anyone to send themselves."[361] And that will remain true even when wireless "virtual reality" technology will sooner or later enable us to hear, see, taste, smell, and feel at a distance.

Thus the atmosphere of a house varies with its occupants.[362] Many persons are able to perceive it optically: in this connection, a Chinese of our own days relates of his father DUN-TSR:

> *He saw with perfect clarity the unavoidable ruin of his family approaching. He even thought he could recognize it in external signs. He was deeply serious when he told me afterward: "When I stood on the wall of the village near the south gate, I saw clearly that the air over our house was dark,*

---

[358]GEORG, Dr. Eugen, *Verschollene Kulturen* [Forgotten Cultures] (Leipzig, 1930), p. 254.
[359]HUEBNER, Dr. Frieder. Mark, *Neimand ist einsam* [No one is isolated] (Kampen/Sylt, 1936), p. 10.
[360]RIESS, Curt, "Goebbels ohne Maske" [Goebbels Unmasked] *die Straße* (1949): 7.
[361]FANKHAUSER, Dr. Alfred, *Magie: Versuch einer astrologischen Lebensdeutung* [Magic: Testing an Astrological Life-Reading] (Zürich, 1934), p. 181 f.
[362]DRESSER, p. 39 f.

but over the west-end family it was bright. It was the will of Heaven."[363]

MEYRINK knew, as hardly any poet before him has known, how to depict individuality in houses.[364] He even ventures to "dream": "That secretly they are the real lords of the alleys, who divest themselves of their life and emotions but can resume them again—in the daytime they lend them to their occupants, only to take them back with interest at nightfall."[365] In aggregate, houses form the village or town. And the atmosphere of the latter also varies according to the nature of its residents.[362] "There are certain mental dowsers who, on entering a locality, can definitely tell whether the prevailing tone of the place is good or bad."[366]

It is a Tibetan belief that Earth's atmosphere is injured by unkind thoughts. Therefore: "foreign visits usually create great difficulties for the Tibetan authorities. The population seems to be convinced that white people send out bad thoughts which gather themselves together, just as water vapor condenses into rain, and fall down on the Tibetans in the form of diseases."[367] Similar views were current in China[368] and were postulated by the Paracelsist Alexander VON SUCHTEN in his *De tribus facultatibus* (ca. 1600). However it is surprising to find them in IMMERMANN:

Is it so preposterous to suppose . . . , that the soul for her part—as the most highly penetrating fluid (? Agens)—exercises an influence on the external world and, in her strongest

---

[363]HWANG TSU-YÜ, *Der blühende Granatapfelbaum* [The Flowering Pomegranate Tree] (Munich, 1948), p. 153.

[364]Meyrink, Gustav, *Des deutschen Spießers Wunderhorn* [Popular Lyrics for the German Commoner], Die Pflanzen des Dr. Cinderella, (Munich and Leipzig, 1948), pp. 237–238.

[365]*Der Golem* (Bremen, 1915), p. 44.

[362]See earlier footnote, page 123.

[366]SCHWARZ, Georg, *Tage und Stunden aus dem Leben eines leutseligen, gottfröhlichen Menschenfreundes, der Johann Friedrich Flattich hieß* [Days and Hours in the Life of an Affable, Bright, and Religious Philanthropist Called Johann Friedrich Flattich] (Tübingen and Stuttgart, 1940), p. 189; STRAUSS-SURYA, pp. 93–94.

[367]NOLLING, T. (Illion, Theod.), "Auf dem Dach der Welt" [On the Roof of the World], *Rhein-Mainische Ztg* (1944), 38 [Feb. 8]: 3.

[368]v. WEISS, J. B., *Weltgeschichte* [World History] vol. I (Vienna and Graz, 1928), p. 69; SCHRÖDTER, Willy, "Wetterzauber" [Weather Magic], *Okk. Stimme* (1954), 7 & 8: 22 f.; STERNEDER, *Frühling im Dorf* [Spring in the Village[, pp. 136–137.

manifestations, is able to impregnate the earth in an analogous way? If one will reason logically and not remain satisfied with half-truths, it is hardly possible to think otherwise. Admittedly, at the present time it can only be put forward as a hypothesis that good people make the earth and the air healthy, whereas evil people pollute them so much that the virtuous shudder, and the weak are tempted to do wrong. This still sounds crazy and baroque, but perhaps in a hundred years it will have become a trivial piece of knowledge.[369]

---

[369]VON FEUCHTERSLEBEN, Dr. Ernst, *Zur Diätetik der Seele* [Mental Dietetics] (Halle/S; Herm. Gesenius, 1910); pp. 15–16.

IDEAS AWAIT
AN EMBODIER

In our own times one cannot pass over in silence "Master
PHILIPPE" *of Lyons, whose reputation was a European one.*
—RIJNBERK *(p. 113)*

On August 2, 1905, 56-year-old Nizier-Anthèlme PHILIPPE died in
his fortress-like villa near Lyons. Under the name "Master
Philippe" he was further known as a thaumaturge. Physicians
like his son-in-law Dr. Emmanuel Henri LALANDE ("Marc Haven,"
1868–1926) and his pupil, the Parisian gynaecologist Dr. Gérard
Anaclet Vincent ENCAUSSE ("Papus," 1865–1926), and important
people like the evangelical esotericist SÉDIR bore witness to his
miraculous cures. ENCAUSSE-PAPUS called him his *maître spirituel*
["spiritual master"] and named his son, who is today practicing
as a doctor in Paris, Philippe for him.[370] As his *maître intellectuel*
PAPUS-ENCAUSSE designated the Marquis SAINT-YVES D'ALVEYDRE,
whom we have mentioned elsewhere.

One day the following took place: A medical commission
consisting of Prof. Camille Hippolyte BROUARDEL (1837–1906),
then chairman of the Medical Faculty of Paris, and the above-
mentioned physicians LALANDE and ENCAUSSE, arrived in the rue
de la Tête d'Or where the thaumaturge worked. With his usual
forcefulness, BROUARDEL explained why they had come, and
PHILIPPE left the choice of patient to him. The commission selected
a lady who was enormously swollen with dropsy and appeared
to be *in extremis.*

Her legs were like pillars, her trunk was like a tower, and her
arms were like Provençal gourds. She seemed ready to burst then

---

[370]SÉDIR, Paul, *Quelques Amis de Dieu* [Some Friends of God] (Bihorel-lez-Rouen, S.I., 1923),
Chapter, "An Unknown," pp. 113–132.

and there . . . the lady was placed on a low stool. "You are here," said PHILIPPE to the commission, and asked, "Can you see okay? . . . Now then . . . that's happened . . ." The lady's skirt had fallen down and was piled around the ankles of the miracle healer. . . . The dropsical patient found herself naked but slim and healed. *There was not a drop of liquid to be seen under the stool or anywhere else.* . . . Was it a miracle? Oh yes, there is no other word for it. A miracle in all its incomprehensible simplicity.

Dr. ENCAUSSE and Dr. LALANDE immediately wrote an official report in which they stated that they had examined the patient before and after and had never taken their eyes off her for a moment; that they were necessarily convinced of the reality of the healing, and that, as a matter of fact, such healings were commonplace with PHILIPPE. . . . They both signed the report, but Prof. BROUARDEL, without denying the event, which would have been very hard to do, refused to add his signature to the two others, on the pretext that *he did not understand what had gone on.*[371]

However, we must not condemn the university doctor too hastily! Even PHILIPPE did not understand himself. "I know nothing at all about myself. I have never understood the mystery that is me and have (also) never tried to explain it to myself. I have performed miraculous cures for the past thirteen years. I am an involuntary middleman between human beings and a power that resides beyond this plane of being. The astounding results I obtain every mortal day fill me with admiration—but I do not comprehend them."

PHILIPPE was just one of those "highly developed individuals" (LAO TSZE; 604–514 [?]), called by the Apostle PAUL "stewards of the mysteries of God"[372] and by PARACELSUS "ministers of Christ," which presumes that just such a "peak human being" is

---

[371]ENCAUSSE, *Le Maître Philippe de Lyon. Thaumaturge et homme de Dieu. Ses prodiges, ses guérisons, ses enseignements* [Master Philippe of Lyons: Thaumaturge and Man of God— His Miracles, His Cures, and His Teachings], IVth ed. (Paris, 1955), p. 81, BOULANGER, Sylvestre, "Ceux qui guérissent et ceux qui tuent" [Those Who Heal and Those Who Kill,] *France au combat* (1948), May 31; BRICAUD, Joanny, *Le Maître Philippe* (Paris); DE ROCHAS, Alb., *Die Ausscheidung des Empfindungs-vermögens* [The Transference of Sensitivity] (Leipzig, 1909), pp. 346–347; DE SAINT-MARTIN, Michel, *Révélations (Entretiens spirituels sur le Maître Philippe de Lyon)* [Revelations (Spiritual talks on Master Philippe of Lyons)]. (Paris: Ed. Psyché, 1938).
[372]I Corinthians 4: 1.

what God wants people to be! Even today, those in search of healing still make a pilgrimage to PHILIPPE's grave in the Loyasse cemetery in Lyons, just as others do to the memorial obelisk of *Paracelsus* in the *Philippo-Neri* chapel in the Church of St. Sebastian, Salzburg!

The "Philippe phenomenon" forms a good introduction to a letter dated August 1, 1958 in which one of those deep-thinking "dwellers in the land"[373] expressed his agreement with my musings on influencing people through one's presence: "All individuals act on one another through their mere presence, but *reciprocally* and within the usual limits. Therefore it seems perfectly natural and attracts absolutely no attention. This interplay is as much a part of life as our daily bread.

However, when people have you in mind, something extraordinary and strange supervenes in a good or bad sense!

There are (discerning and humble) impersonal people, and others who, because of some fixed idea (ambition, lust for power, lasciviousness), are bereft of personality.[374]

Ordinary human interplay ceases in the presence of either of these, because the *human* partner is missing!

One is unexpectedly brought up against the SUPER-human or the IN-human and feels its presence even if one's thinking brain is unaware of it. The Maoris call it *mana*.[375]

It is perceptible as a *non-specific* force present behind the silence and self-emptying of the sages, and creates a distance around them at the same time. With the sages, we warm ourselves at it without being burned. On the other hand, someone who is devoid of personality is a "Trojan horse" used by *specific* forces, which so obliterate him that they become a *person*[376] in

---

[373]Psalm 37: 3.

[374]The term "impersonal" for unselfish people strikes me as better than HUCH's "bereft of personality" (loc. cit.).

[375]This word was brought back from Polynesia by the English missionary CODRINGTON, who was the first to write about mystical power. The Australian aborigines speak of *Yoia* and the Sioux use the expression *Wakantanka*. (TENHAEFF, pp. 233–234).

[376]Cf. the expression, "He is all stomach, or "whose god is their belly" (Philippians 3: 19), or, "all he is made of is food and drink." Dr. Andreas Justinus Christian KERNER (1786–1862) wrote to Sophie SCHWAB on April 12, 1836 that, "Some people have the minds of sows. When their body fails, the sow or *sow spirit* emerges, looking like a sow and visible to those who can see ghosts." ANGELUS SILESIUS (*The Cherubic Wanderer*) said, "A person

him and, through this breach, burst in on our human world. And then we confront the *personified* vice, etc. as something inhuman and disturbing.[377]

In some such way we may account for the surpassing all human measure by such exponents, their mysterious influence, and their immunity to human feeling.[378] When they are fundamentally unsound, they fall, and invariably recognize too late that they have been deceived deceivers!

Active sex-bombs—including the *Don Juans*[379]—are also Trojan horses of this sort. The *passive sex bombs* are attractive hollow forms, sexually frigid, but exerting the powerful suction of a sexual vacuum on either sex.

As a natural phenomenon, they are also impersonal, and therefore a grave for personified passions. The (impersonal) *healer* usually has no inkling of the true state of affairs! The

---

who indulges the appetites like a brute beast is only a hollow mask, appearing to be something, yet actually nothing." In this connection I cannot refrain from reproducing—certainly to the joy of many—the observation of an old mesmerist. In the *Jahrbüchern für den Lebens-Magnetismus oder Neues Askläpieion* (Leipzig, 1819), II Bd., 2: 1–16, under the heading "Mesmerthum und Arzneikram" [Mesmerism and Medical Matters] a certain Dr. Riecke (of Stuttgart) made the following remarks: "Nevertheless the animal with which a person habitually lives has a strong influence on his character. The Tartar, who is a horseman, has something equine about him; the shepherd is placid; the swine-herd is piggy; the goose-girl is silly; and the Greenlander, who sees nothing but seals, becomes like a seal in body and soul." The last statement is illustrated by the photograph I have in front of me, as I write, of the over 70-year-old Eskimo *Kungeyuak* from East Greenland, whose rescue work is featured in the book *Notlandung* [Emergency Landing] by the Danish poet Erling Poulsen (Hamann-Meyerpress). This book won a prize offered by the Association of Scandinavian authors. Then there was keeper *Nulpe*, at Hagenbeck's zoo in Hamburg-Stellingen, who over the years came to look more and more like his pet seal "Barry."

[377]Dr. Huebner (of Amsterdam) calls this an "irrational fulness of being." Dr. Erwin Liek discusses its good side in his *Das Wunder in der Heilkunde* [The Miraculous in Therapeutics] (Munich, 1930), p. 194.

[378]Elisha (850 B.C.) the successor of Elijah, asked for a double portion of the latter's spirit (II Kings 2: 9). This "spirit-grafting" (Hebrew: *Ibbur*) took place. Elisha underwent a complete transformation into *Elijahu*, and just as the latter in his capacity as the earthly vessel of Yahweh was not subject to human sentiment (II Kings 1: 10, 12), so the same was true of Elisha (II Kings 2: 23–24), because he was "possessed" by the spirit of Elijah. Significantly, the spirit of Elijah came upon his helper after the latter had taken up Elijah's mantle (II Kings 2: 13). This was not so much a symbol of protective covering as of a "transference of Od" (I Kings 19: 19).

[379]Kästner, Erich, "Es gibt noch Don Juans" [Don Juans are Still With Us], *Berl. Tagebl.* (1930), February 21, morning edition; Lermontow, Michail Jurjewitsch, "Ein Held unsere Zeit" [A Hero of Our Times], *Reclam* 968–969, p. 117.

"virtue" (PARACELSUS) clings to him or her just as flavor clings to the camomile. If a spirit of pride tempts him or her to try and work out how "he" or "she" produces "it," the magic vanishes, for it is the "it" that makes "him" or "her" what he or she is.

Actually there are no "radiators of healing," but only superior "reflectors"[380] and "convergent lenses" for nature's inherent power of regeneration.[381] Obviously these convergent lenses are human beings who are in a special state of selflessness (we are not referring here to benevolence, generosity, etc.) involving attraction and permeability. They are rather like a ventilator that thrusts and so creates a vacuum, which drags everything toward it and makes possible an endless inflow and through-flow until it gets stuck (starts clinging to self) and then stops, whereby success becomes impossible. And this is what happens to those healers who rise like comets and then start boasting of their powers and "strike an attitude," only to vanish into a memory.

---

[380]Cf. the "telepathic mirror," (*Walpurgisnacht* (1917), p. 15, 113 f. of MEYRINK, the actor *Zrcadlo* (Czech: "mirror").

[381]Jean BÉZIAT, the miracle healer of Avignonet (Haute-Garonne) used to appeal to "Great Nature" when he was performing miraculous cures and also evoked the aid of "all good spirits in God's service" (Dr. Jean VINCENT, *Les Révélations des Guérisseurs* [Revelations of the Healers] (Paris-Bernhardin-Béchet, 1931), pp. 98–99; Also the magneto-magist Antonio REGAZZONI of Bergamo (died in 1870), in whom SCHOPENHAUER took an interest, confessed: "I include a little invocation in all my difficult operations, but only to benign spirits." (DES MOUSSEAUX: *La Magie au XIXe siècle* [Magic in the 19th Century] (1860), p. 247; A. J. RIKO, *Handbuch zur Ausübung des Magnetismus, des Hypnotismus, der Suggestion, der Biologie und verwandter Fächer* [A Practical Handbook of Mesmerism, Hypnotism, Suggestion, Biology, and Related Matters] (Leipzig, 1904), p. 143; Evidently, to some extent, BÉZIAT was what we should call today a "spiritual healer"! It is not widely known that, long before English spiritual healers visited us after World War II, one of great ability had been active here in Germany for several years. It was this man, the "miracle doctor of Homburg" (Bad Homburg v.d. H.), Gustav Adolf MÜLLER-CZERNY (1862–1922) who later adopted the forenames "Egmont" and "Roderich." The latter because he claimed that "*Roderich of Bern*" stood behind him in a column of helpers in the shape of "ultraviolet entities." (Dr. Herm. HAUPT, *Die strahlende Lebenskraft und ihr Gesetze* [The Radiating Life Force and Its Laws] (Althofnaß bei Breslau, 1922), pp. 91–92; This is no other than "*Berndietrich*," *Dietrich von Bern* (Verona), the *Thidrek* of the Nordic sagas. He appears mainly in the *Thidrek Saga*, the *Hildebrandlied* and the *Nibelungenlied* and has a historical counterpart in the Ostrogoth king *Theoderich the Great* (454/471/526). "I do not impose anything, nor do I even propose anything, I expose"—in connection with which the philanthropic instincts of the ex-journalist MÜLLER were a great credit to him: he supported 50 orphans and 21 families.

"Subud," like "Abu-Bekr-Zikr" are meant to do nothing more than to create the vacuum.[382] If it occurs—if the exercise is performed in the right spirit—then the proper forces must come into play, for *nature abhors a vacuum!*[383]

Of course this makes the worldling very fearful, because a new situation dawns which has never been experienced before and initially leaves him or her feeling quite helpless."[384]

Zikr means "recollection"; there are two types of this exercise, which are said to keep awake the memory of the "soul's homeland of Light." *Abu-Bekr-Zikr* is the silent exercise of the Nakshi-bendi Dervishes: it is called *Ali-Zikr* however.

---

[382] ANGELUS SILESIUS: "The more you can put off / yourself and pour it out, / the more will God flow in / to you beyond all doubt." Complete self-emptying—the death of self—is the secret of the art of archery in Zen Buddhism. When this *conditio sine qua non* is fulfilled, the IT presses into the vacated ego-space, and the IT shoots and always hits the target. (Prof. Karl DÜRCKHEIM, *The Japanese and the Culture of Tranquility*. Prof. Eugen HERRIGEL: *Zen in the Art of Archery*).

[383] A Rosicrucian axiom, carved on the altar gravestone of Christian ROSENCREUTZ (1378–1484). The metaphysical equivalent of this physical law of the *horror vacui* (Latin for: "horror of empty space") is finely expressed by Jeanne Marie Bouvières de la Mothe GUYON (1648–1717) in her *Moyen court de faire oraison* [Short and Easy Method of Prayer]: "As soon as we esteem ourselves as nothing, God, who does not and cannot leave any emptiness unfilled, must flow into us."

[384] A case in point is that of the Danish Anthroposophist Director Carl VETT (1871–1956) who in his *Seltsamen Erlebnissen in einem Derwischkloster* [Strange Experiences in a Dervish Monastery] (Straßburg: Heitz & Co., 1931), p. 183, offers a far-fetched description of a controversy with the Dervishes which (it is painfully obvious) is nothing more than a cover-up for his withdrawal. He pulled out because of panic over the impending "sinking into a state of non-modality" (MEISTER ECKEHART; 1260–1327). He wanted to *"com*-prehend" but not to be *"ap*-prehended"!

ON BEING
USED BY GOD ...

And of this I am quite conscious: that God's creative and renewing power flows through my whole being like incoming waves of electricity.

—*Dr. Toyochiko* KAGAWA

We have seen that remarkable cures—including the instant dispersal of the most serious diseases, even from a distance—take place through certain individuals who have become impersonal. It would be childish to ascribe such therapeutic successes to the human "transmitters," who are no more than the "relay stations" of a "higher power." That this is so is made absolutely clear by the well-known telephone cures of humans and animals bitten by the deadly priskok (spring viper) which, with Allah's help, have been performed free of charge since 1901 by Mustapha Effendi MUJAGITSCH of Sarajevo (born in 1875). The healing formula of evocation has been handed down for 300 years in the highly respected family of this Finance Ministry auditor, now retired—a deeply devout Moslem, educated at Turkish, Arabian, and Persian schools, whom I visited on July 11, 1955: it was the princely gift of an itinerant sheikh of the *Rufai Dervishes,* to whom a great service had been rendered.[385] The celebrated Swiss psychologist

---

[385]BECKES, Theodor, "Die Schlangenkönige von Bosnien" [The Snake King of Bosnia], *Berl. Tagebl.* (1937), Dec. 31, Extract from supplement "Mustapha Effendi heilt auch telefonisch" [Mustapha Effendi Also Heals Over the Phone]; SACHER-MASOCH, Alexander, "Jenseits der osmanischen Grenze, Streiflichter einer zaubervollen Balkanfahrt" [Over the Ottoman Border, Side-Lights on a Magical Balkan Tour], *Basler National-Ztg* (1954), Sept 26, reprinted under the caption "Mustapha Effendi Mujagitsch, Heilung durchs Telefon" [Mustapha Effendi Mujagitsch, Healing by Phone], *Neue Wiss.* (1954), 11–12 [Nov./Dec.]: 374 f.; Dr. B. JACOBSON, once again: "Healing by Telephone," *Neue Wiss.* (1955), 5–6 [May–June]: 186 f.; MAREIS, Dr. Ingo, "Reise in die Vergangenheit" [A Journey Into the Past], *Der Fackelreiter* (1955), June 2 No., extract from "Heilung durch das Telefon"; SCHRÖDTER, Willy, "Zu Besuch bei dem Heiler Mustapha Mujagitsch" [A Visit to the Healer Mustapha Mujagitsch, *Neue Wiss.* (1955), 11–12 [Nov.–Dec.]: 371.

Dr. Hugo DEBRUNNER (born in 1895) has verified the gift of distant healing possessed by this deeply pious man, and has found unusual line formations on his hands and feet (and also on his two sisters SULEIKA and REIFKA). All the hand-lines flow to the thumb but stop just before they reach it. Dr. DEBRUNNER interprets this as "a flow into the All," and, in this connection, suggests that the unconscious of the medium is able to form a link, as it were, with the other world.[386]

M. had extraordinary teachers: in the *Öffentlichen Anzeiger f.d. Kreis Krueznach* (No. 168 of July 20, 1944, 2) we read under the caption: "*I am going to die on June 20, 1944.*"

"Belgrade July 20. The mullah TAZKO has died in Sarajevo. His death has created quite a stir, chiefly because he prophesied it. Several years ago he procured a gravestone and had inscribed on it: 'Died on June 20, 1944 at 12 noon.' And in fact his death did occur on June 20 at midday. What is more it was a natural death from old age."

In reply to my inquiry of January 7, 1956, my fatherly friend wrote to me on the 23rd of the same month: "What you have read is true. He was our great teacher, who called himself Hadshi Hafiz Shakir Effendi TUZLO, my dear and unforgettable teacher, who lived long. His son is now a professor at the gymnasium."

Also the saintly sheikh (marabout) of the family OULED SIDI BÉNAMAR in the Néroma district (Dép: Oran; Arr.: Tlemcen)— bearing the name SIDI MOULAY ALI BEN LARDI BÉNAMAR—heals theurgically (in addition to certain types of sciatica) the bites of poisonous and rabid animals, even from a distance. Not only members of the indigenous population, but also the French— even from France itself, including people from the upper stratum of society—consult the miracle healer. In the same way as before, the vehicle is a secret formula handed down from father to the most worthy son for hundreds of years (Yahia Boutemène, *La Zaouia des Ouled Sidi Bénamar près de Néroma*. Tlemcen o. J. [after 1941]). The use of the word "vehicle" and not "agent" is deliberate. I use "vehicle" for the call that evokes transcendental forces—which is what I believe happens.

---

[386]ANONYMOUS, "Geisterspuk unter der Forscherlupe" [Spooks Under the Magnifying Glass], (VII), *Heim u. Welt* (1957), 16 [April 19], 8th section "Erlebnis in Jugoslawien" [An Adventure in Yugoslavia].

MUJAGITSCH, with whom I shared this in my letter of May 1, 1957, replied as follows on May 8, 1957: "Among the Moslems in East Asia and Africa there are still many learned and very learned men known by name, who are working like SIDI MOULAY ALI BEN LARDI. I have some more written proofs. You are welcome to come back here so that I can show them to you!" The words of the over 70-year-old Dervish, Hadji Ahmad al TABRIZI of Kerind (in Northern Iran) apply to all these Moslem healers: "You ask me the secret of the true dervish. I say that it is surrender to the Will of God. . . . The man who does not surrender to God's Will becomes inevitably the slave of this world, and cannot escape from it even if he unceasingly calls upon the name of God" (Bennett, p. 48).

There are also some European miracle healers: Cyprien VIGNES (died in 1908) of Vialas (Lozère) had the gift of curing the incurable from a distance. When asked for the secret of his healings, he replied: "It's quite simple, I see the Lord beside me and He tells me what to do and say, and He Himself does the healing" (Gg. SULZER, *Die Bedeutung der Wissenschaft vom Übersinnlichen für Bibel und Christentum*).

Then there is the clairvoyant peasant Josef HILDWEIN (died ca. 1930) of Wollmannsberg bei Stockerau (near Vienna), who used prayer in addition to animal magnetism. Hanging on the walls of his waiting room were certificated framed letters from several Viennese doctors and professors, or members of their families, whom he had freed from serious diseases. SURYA was permitted to observe him at work over a period of three weeks in 1898. A remarkable circumstance was that if anyone tried to dupe him, the thought-reading healer could fly into a rage, but would lose his clairvoyant gift for three days owing to his wasteful expenditure of emotions (SURYA, *Okkulte Diagnostik u. Prognostik* [Occult Diagnosis and Prognosis], Lorch I. W., 1950, pp.20–22, 199).

Finally, perhaps we should add Léon ALALOUF (born 1905), now living in Toulouse, who heals not only by the laying on of hands, but also from a distance, and infallibly picks out the most urgent cases from his daily sackful of mail. At all events his celebrated advocate, the attorney Dr. MORO-GIAFERI (born 1872) declared in court that he owed his energy to ALALOUF, and at another hearing in Paris in 1950, the latter healed by touch (at the request of the president of the tribunal) one of the jurors who was suffering in agony from sciatica.

With reference to such miracle cures, which defy any parapsychological explanation, Taoism, that most abstract of religions would say: Miracle cures of this kind are performed by "superior people" who have unified their "human Tao" with the "Tao of heaven," people who are not swimming against the stream, but who resign themselves to being borne along by it (the Christian "rule," *Wu-Wei*). "Being the most unselfish of all, he [the Master] endures and fulfils his primary purpose." (*Tao-Têh King*, VII). [Translation taken from *The Simple Way of Lao Tsze*, London, The Shrine of Wisdom, 1924, p. 19. *Tr.*]. CHRIST says exactly the same (Luke 17: 33 ["Whosoever shall seek to save his life shall lose it; and whosoever shall lose his life shall preserve it."]) in His teaching concerning a personal God: "I seek not mine own will, but the will of the Father which hath sent me" (John 5: 30). "The Father that dwelleth in me, he doeth the works" (John: 14: 10). To be a follower, the disciple of Christ must deny himself or herself (Matthew 16: 24 ["If any man will come after me, let him deny himself, and take up his cross and follow me."]), which is like a crucifixion to the "love of self."

METANOIA

Thus the lesson is this, that it is necessary to make a *metanoia* (Greek: "change of mind") of 180° involving putting a love of one's neighbor above self-love. This was a primary requirement of the Essene [?] ascetic JOHN THE BAPTIST (Matthew 3: 2—["Repent ye—*metanoeite*—for the kingdom of heaven is at hand"]), and after him of the LORD himself (Matthew 4: 17 ["Repent—*metanoeite*—for the kingdom of heaven is at hand."]). Among the "signs" flowing from such dedication are healing by the laying on of hands (Mark 16: 17–18 ["And these signs shall follow them that believe: in my name . . . they shall lay hands on the sick, and they shall recover."]). The Apostle PAUL terms them "spiritual gifts" (Greek: [*pneumatika* and] *charismata*; I Corinthians 12). Indian Yoga has its *siddhi*.

Prayer and Fasting

On one occasion the disciples of JESUS were unable to cast out the spirit of disease in a severe case of "moon-madness" (epilepsy) (Matthew 17: 14–21). At that time certain diseases were recognized as entities (Luke 4: 39 ["And he stood over her, and rebuked the fever; and it left her"]), just as in Islamic *Tarikaat*[387] today, or in some contemporary Western medical authors, many mental disorders associated with an otherwise intact brain are seen as caused by, and in need of treatment as, possession (Latin: *possessio*).

Examples of such authors are the often mentioned Dr. Franz HARTMANN, also Dr. Carl D. ISENBERG (1876–1941) and, above all, Dr. Carl A. WICKLAND (1862–1937) of Los Angeles.[388]

In answer to the question "Why could not we cast him out?" asked by those who had already been empowered to cast out unclean spirits and to "heal all manner of disease" (Matthew 10: 1), the Lord said, among other things: "Howbeit this kind goeth not out but by *prayer* and *fasting*" [Matthew 17:21].

Since these words—rightly understood—contain the whole way of hallowing and healing (and also of being a healer), we need to take a look at them, however briefly.

What is meant by "prayer" is obviously not the repeated recitation of standard ready-made prayers (Matthew 6: 7 ["Use not vain repetitions"]), but a continual resort to prayer (Luke 18: 1 ["Men ought always to pray, and not to faint"]). It is the "praying without ceasing" (Greek: *adialeiptos*) spoken of by the Apostle PAUL (I Thessalonians 5: 17), and his daily "supplication in the spirit" to God (Ephesians 6: 18). It is the "practice of the presence of God"[389] as performed during a long life by the French Carmelite, Brother Lawrence (Nicholas HERMANN, 1610–1691), which the mystic Gerhard TERSTEGEN (1697–1769) enlarged on in

[387]VETT, p. 284.
[388]WICKLAND, Carl A., *Thirty Years Among the Dead*, in collaboration with Nella M. WATTS, Celia L. GOERTZ, Orland D. GOERTZ (Los Angeles: Nat. Psychol. Inst. 1924).
[389]LORENZ, Ernst, *Die Vergegenwärtigung Gottes im praktischen Leben: Gespräche und Briefe von Bruder Laurentius* [The Practice of the Presence of God in Daily Life: The Discourses and Letters of Brother Lawrence]. (Bad Pyrmont, n.d.)

Wuppertal: "We must our piety and godliness into the kitchen, into the field, and anywhere we have occasion to go. We should and must serve God in all places and in everything we do."

The black American genius (Acts 10: 34–35) Dr. George Washington CARVER (1864–1943) used to go into the forest in the early hours (Mark 1: 35 ["And in the morning, rising up a great while before day, he went out, and departed into a solitary place and there prayed."]; Proverbs 8: 17 ["Those that seek me early shall find me."]) to commune with his "dear Creator," and had revealed to him the secrets of the peanut[390] and the sweet potato[391] not to mention his rediscovery of an Ancient Egyptian fast dye of exceptional brilliance.[392]

Such condescension by God to us and our earthly concerns can take place only on our simple level. The saintly curé of Ars-en-Dombes (Ain), Jean-Baptiste Marie VIANNEY (1786–1859) set down as the sum total of his practical experience: "Faith means speaking to God as one would to another person."[393]

Fasting can mean abstaining from food. We understand by this more than a temporary loss of appetite (Exodus 34: 28 ["And he was there with the LORD forty days and forty nights; he did neither eat bread, nor drink water.]; I Kings 19: 8 ["And he arose, and did eat and drink, and went in the strength of that meat forty days and forty nights."]; Matthew 4: 2 ["And when he had fasted forty days and forty nights, he was afterward an hungered."]). The therapeutic and character-building effects of fasting need not be discussed any further here.

Another point to consider is "civilization asceticism," or abstention from non-essentials, which is the only course still open to us if we are not to end up as the playthings of a consumer society.[394] The danger—to speak in Paracelsian terms—of be-

---

[390]CLARK, Dr. Clenn, *Der Mann, der mit den Blumen spricht. Die Lebensgeschichte Dr. George Washington Carvers, von einem Freunde erzählt* [The Man Who Converses with Flowers: The Life Story of Dr. George Washington Carver Told by a Friend] (Bad Pyrmont, 1950), p. 49.
[391]CLARK, p. 21.
[392]CLARK, pp. 26–27; HOLT, Rackham, *Der Pflanzendoktor George Washington Carver* [The Botanical Doctor, George Washington Carver] (Munich, Leipzig, Freiburg i. B., 1949).
[393]SÉDIR, *Quelques Amis* [A Few Friends], p. 98; DE FABREGUES, Jean, *J. M. Vianney, der Zeuge von Ars* [J. M. Vianney, The Witness of Ars] (Freiburg, i. Br., n.d.).
[394]BODAMER, Dr. Joachim, "Der Mensch ohne Ich" [People Without Individuality], *Herder-Bücherei* (1958), No. 21.

coming immersed in things (or activities) or, to put it another way, of being turned into a "thing" and being compelled to serve one's own things (!) has been present *in potentia* from the very beginning. Life is now not only physically perilous, it is also detrimental to the soul. "What shall it profit a man, if he shall gain the whole world, and lose his own soul?" (Mark 8: 36), asks CHRIST; and he warns us against over-valuing physical comfort (Matthew 6: 25 ["Is not the life more than meat, and the body more than raiment?"]). The Apostle PAUL, too, advised us to limit ourselves to the necessities (I Timothy 6: 6–8 ["Godliness with contentment is great gain . . . having food and raiment let us be therewith content"]); and LAO TSZE knew how possessions could possess their possessor (at least during the latter's lifetime).[395] To sum up in the words of Garcia LORCA: "The fewer earthly things one takes to be important, the nearer one comes to really important things."

Being sparing with our words—word fasting—by which we mean refraining from every unnecessary and unprofitable utterance (as an exercise in self-control, and *not* due to laziness) is equally important. As Prof. MATTHIAS[330] says, silence has its virtues: deliberate word asceticism strengthens the will, deepens the thoughts, and increases their power of penetration. Indeed, SCHOPENHAUER may be taken to underpin this philosophically: the "will to live" feels threatened or inhibited by abstention, on the denser planes, from one of its major activities (in this case "talking"), and by dint of its metaphysical identity, creates an equalization on a subtle plane.[396]

The "Word" himself (John 1: 14 ["And the Word was made flesh, and dwelt among us"]) has indicated in an alarming way

---

[395]LAO TSZE: *Tao-Têh King XII* ["A diversity of light tends to blind the eyes. A diversity of sounds tends to deafen the ears. A diversity of flavours tends to dull the taste. A diversity of actions tends to excite the desires. A diversity of quests tends to corrupt the intentions. That is why the self-controlled man closes the doors of the senses and dwells in the inner Life." Loc. cit. p. 50. *Tr.*].

[330]See earlier footnote, page 113.

[396]SCHRÖDTER, Willy, *Streifzug ins Ungewohnte* [An Excursion into the Unusual] (Freiburg i. Br., 1949), see the chapter on silence, p. 97; and "Lieber Sweigen als Reden" [It is Better to be Silent Than to Speak], *Psychol. Mh.* (1958), No. XII), p. 351 f.

(Matthew 12: 36 ["Every idle word that men shall speak, they shall give account thereof in the day of judgment."]) the metaphysical background of the import of the spoken word. The discipline of silence rightly belongs to the primordial observances of genuine "occult" secret societies and to many monastic orders such as the *Trappists*.

SILENCE THERAPY

For the cure or, at least, for the alleviation of certain diseases, a "silence therapy" has been available for some time now. It was originated by Heinrich JÜRGENS,[397] and then carried on by Hossein Kazemzadeh IRANSCHÄR[398] and more recently by Dr. Betty FISHER (Philadelphia). The findings of modern medical science suggest that we ought not to say that people talk too much because they are nervy, but should rather say that too much talking is giving them an adverse nervous deficit! The Greek physician Dr. Ari TSAGALOS has given the name *logodiarrhea* to this pathological prodigality of words. The well-known psychologist, Dr. Gert MICHAEL, advocates "days of silence" by saying "noisy motors don't work."[399]

"THROUGH GOD WE SHALL DO VALIANTLY" (PSALM 60: 12)

It is possible to construct the systematics of a Christian *theurgy* (Psalm 60: 12) as follows: "God is love / and he that dwelleth in love / dwelleth in God / and God in him." (I John 4: 16). Again it is written: "He that abideth in me / and I in him / the same

---

[397]JÜRGENS, Heinrich, *Schweige dich gesund!* [Get Well by Being Silent!] (Pfullingen i. W., 1922).

[398]KAZEMZADEH-IRANSCHÄR, H., *Die Heilkraft des Schweigens* [The Healing Power of Silence], 4th ed. (Zürich, 1948).

[399]MICHAEL, Dr. Gert, "Halte den Mund, schweig dich gesund!" [Hold Your Tongue and Get Well Through Silence], *Heim u. Welt* (1955), 18 [May 4]: 1, 11.

bringeth forth much fruit / for without me ye can do nothing."
(John 15: 5). The "fruit" are the "signs" related by MARK.

One could spin the thread further: ". . . that by these ye
might be partakers of the divine nature, having escaped the cor-
ruption that is in the world through lust" (II Peter 1: 4), and "For
our conversation [or "citizenship"] is in heaven; from whence
also we look for the Saviour, the Lord JESUS CHRIST: who shall
change our vile body, that it may be fashioned like unto his glori-
ous body, according to the working whereby he is able even to
subdue all things unto himself" (Philippians 3: 20–21).

The "Silesian nightingale" made a poetic translation of
Peter's sentence: "If you outgrow yourself / and all the creatures,
Implanted you will find / God's wondrous features."

But the idea that love, or unlimited goodwill, or altruism is
the therapeutic agent, is encountered in all zones and in every
age.[95]

MAN SHALL NOT LIVE BY BREAD ALONE . . .

An old story will serve to show that human beings do not live by
bread alone (Matthew 4: 4) and that, for example, mother love is
"the vitamin of the soul," as the British research worker Dr.
BOWLY said to an international congress in 1953. There is an old
story that the Staufer Kaiser FRIEDRICH II (1215–1250) wanted to
find out which was the original human language and decided
that, if a child is not taught to speak, it will reproduce the primitive language of mankind on its own initiative. And so he placed
a number of babies in the care of nurses and gave them strict orders not to speak to their charges. In spite of the fact that the latter were given the best food and the optimum physical care, all
the test subjects went into a decline, because they received no
emotional support from endearments and words of comfort.
They were spiritually "hungry" as the well-known pediatrician
Prof. VON PFAUNDLER called it! (Dr. Heinz GRAUPNER).

---

[95]See earlier note, page 34.

THE SPITZ EFFECT

In 1954 French zoologists confirmed by animal experiments the utility of this emotional support: each morning they spent several minutes affectionately stroking baby rats in their cages. The animals that had been handled with "love" really thrived; their bone structure was stronger than that of rats which had not been stroked. The test was repeated with the same result by WEININGER, a psychologist of German origin living in Canada, using two sets of ten rats, and by Lew BERNSTEIN in Denver, CO using two sets of twenty rats.

A report on the latter was issued by Prof. René A. SPITZ (born 1887) who was appointed Professor of Clinical Psychiatry in the University of Denver, and has functioned as Research Consultant for Child Psychiatry at the Lennox Hill Hospital in New York, and to whom we are indebted for a valuable work on "First-formed object relationships"[400] and who packed his knowledge into the short article "Säuglinge brauchen Liebe" [Babies Need Love].[401] They need love "to cover them as continually and as closely as their own skin," as otherwise they can suffer from organic neuroses. This is the so-called "Spitz effect": a discovery that "each mother can win a smile because she instinctively knows how to do so; she does not need to be taught."[402]

Thus we are certainly not dealing with some purely odic cause, but with the love-drenched aura of the mother that soothes the restless child in her bosom. It is along these lines that Dr. Johann F. OSLANDER (1787–1855) sometime professor of medicine in Göttingen and Waldeck Court Counsellor, writes: "The best way to soothe a restless child is for the mother to take it to bed with her. Old Jacob RUEFF in his days (in Plate XI of a little book titled *Schön lustig Trostbüchle von Empängknussen*, etc." 1554) advises that after the child has been washed and swaddled, it

---

[400]SPITZ, René A., *Die Entstehung der ersten Objektbeziehungen* [First-Formed Object Relationships]. 1937.

[401]GERSTER, Dr. Gg., "Säuglinge brauchen Liebe" [Babies Need Love], from *Die Werkstatt des Wissens*, 2nd edition (Frankfurt/M., 1958), Ullstein-Buch No. 196, p. 129 f.

[402]BODAMER, pp. 67–68.

should be given to the mother in bed '*next to her heart on the left side.*'"[403]

Love means: seeing a person as God has wanted them to be.
—*F.M. Dostojewskij (1821–1881)*

Prince GAUTAMA SIDDHARTA, the Buddha (560–480 B.C.) said: "Nirvana is there, where you are not!" Naturally this does not mean where you no longer are in general, but where you no longer are with your self-centered (egocentric) thinking!

SURYA has shown in detail that this *Nirvana* (= "no more illusion anywhere") is not an annihilation of consciousness but an expansion into "*cosmic* consciousness."[404]

"The enlightened one" says of his *arahat* (he whose journey is accomplished) almost as if referring to a HUTER- or RILLSTROEM-like ethereal radiating force of love: "He radiates a loving spirit in one direction, then in a second, then in a third, then in a fourth, also upwards and downwards; he completely illuminates the whole world with a loving spirit, wide, deep, unbounded, and cleared of rage and malice."

In taking this view, one finds confirmation in another of Buddha's sayings: "Love shines and flames and radiates." The view is also upheld by a specialist in Indian religions: "Since all beings are subject to suffering, the first ethical requirement is compassion and help. *This ethical frame of mind is not only meaningful for the individual but is like a force that goes out of him or her: 'rays of kindness'!*"[405]

This is a good place to recall the legend about the envious Raja DEVADATTA launching a war-elephant against his cousin GAUTAMA. The latter remained sitting in the lotus position, willing

[403]OSIANDER, Joh. F., *Volksarzneimittel und einfache, nicht pharmazeutische Heilmittel gegen Krankheiten des Menschen* [Folk Medicine and Simple Non-Pharmaceutical Remedies for Human Diseases] (Ulm/Donau; Karl F. Haug Verlag, 1957), p. 181 (sub. 10).

[404]SURYA, G. W., *Ursachen der Krankheiten und Wesen des Leides* [The Causes of Disease and the Nature of Suffering] (Lorch i. W., 1937), p. 20 f; BUCKE, Dr. Maurice, *Cosmic Consciousness: A Study in the Evolution of the Human Mind* (Philadelphia, 1901); NIELSEN, pp. 263–264; SCHRÖDTER, Willy, *Abenteuer mit Gedanken* [Adventures with Ideas] (Freiburg i. Br., 1954), see the chapter on "Cosmic Consciousness", pp. 25–26.

[405]ECKERT, Dr. Victor, *Die Geheimlehre* [The Secret Doctrine] (of H. P. Blavatsky), vol. 8 (Berlin, 1958), p. 31.

a stream of love to flow toward the enraged animal, and the latter knelt down in front of him!

Possibly the following Indian proverb goes back to that time: "Good people resemble holy bathing places, for the sight, touch, mention, and memory of them removes all uncleanness."

PARACELSUS (died 1541) in the "Hospital Book," said, "The most important foundation of medicine is love." GOETHE (died 1832) said, "Where a good man treads the place is consecrated." Dr. Arthur LUTZE, Member of the Board of Health (died 1870), said in his *Lehrbuch der Homöopathie*, "Everyone who has visited my clinic has seen that often the most severe pains subside in response to the touch of my hand, my breath, or my bare word. Yes, sometimes, diseases that have lasted for years have suddenly vanished forever. This is a gift of God which cannot be learned by study, and yet—as the facts proclaim—does exist and is dependent on belief and will. I must believe that there really is such a power and that it has been bestowed on me by God Almighty. And when, on the strength of this belief, I have a firm resolve to help my suffering brother, I may do what I will in God's name; that is to say, I may lay on hands, or make a pass or two with them, or just extend them towards the patient, or I may breathe on him, or merely say a word—and his pain will be relieved and his disease will end. When I am unable to help, either it is because my faith is weak, or (and powerfully magnetic people will understand what I mean) something unseen warns me that I am not permitted to help in that particular case."[247]

A favorite saying of the distinguished mesmerist Armand Marie Jacques de Chastenet, Marquis DE PUYSÉGUR (1751–1825) was: "Veuillez et croyez!" [Exercise your will and your faith!]

PARACELSUS said, "You must want to help, and the Spirit of Truth will lead and guide you!"—But what is the pure desire to help, if it is not goodwill or love?

HEIN (p. 68) says: "The Ens Deale of PARACELSUS is the divine decree (Matthew 5: 26 [Verily I say unto thee, Thou shalt by no means come out thence, till thou hast paid the uttermost farthing.])—the Indian *karma*."

---

[247]See earlier footnote page 87.

Helena Petrovna BLAVATSKY (died 1891) reported in *Mysterious Races* that the nomadic *Toda* of the Nilgiri mountains (Southern India) treat their diseases by exposure to the sun's rays and a transfer of vital force, and that one of their elders had declared: "We heal with the love that streams from the sun, but it has no effect on an evil person." This remarkable tribe, which is on the verge of extinction (population 800 in 1901, 474 in 1952) worships 14 gods whose names and forms must have been imported from Babylon.[406]

G. W. SURYA (1907) said, "A good unselfish person has an invigorating and refreshing effect on all beings. In every respect he is a stream of blessing. Wherever he comes, he spreads light and warmth. Broken hearts and minds filled with despair are comforted by his words and look. One feels calm and secure when he is near. This is where I penetrated the secret of successful priests, physicians, and teachers."[407]

"Heliodapath" Carl HUTER (died 1912) said, "I have established that love is the essence of vital, emotional, and radiant force and must be regarded as the maker of all things, for in my radiation experiments the transmissions of *helioda* are prolonged and strengthened by loving thoughts, and they are diminished as these become fewer, and disappear with indifference and unkindness.

"Thus it seems as if the vital rays draw nourishment from a concealed omnipotence which is love, and as if, without love, omnipotence could not, or would not, empower anyone. I have become convinced that this concealed omnipotence is essentially an inexhaustible love and goodness, and the sustainer of all things (of all life and being), and has been here from eternity" (SCHRÖDTER, *Offenbarungen* [Revelations], p. 54).

Christian WAGNER (died 1918) the Swabian peasant poet, has portrayed in a poem in memory of Friedrich RÜCKERT (1788–1866) titled "The Brahmin" how all nature repays him with love because he is a traveling stream of blessing (SURYA; cf. Genesis 12: 2! ["... and thou shalt be a blessing"]:

---

[406]OPPERT, "Über die Toda und Kâta" [The Toda and the Kâta], *Z. Ethnologie* XXVIII, 216.
[407]SURYA: *Rosenkreuzer* [The Rosicrucians], p. 39.

"Where'er he wanders and where'er he treads,
Peace follows him and blessing spreads."

And when we read lower down in the poem:

"The big cats with their panther fur;
They lick his hand, he hears them purr."

We cannot dismiss it as fiction. "Perfect love casteth out fear" (I John 4: 18) as the "beloved" disciple of JESUS could say from personal experience. All wild cats bow before and serpents are tamed by such love. Recent evidence for this is to be found in the reports of the "white yogi" and former London journalist Paul BRUNTON. After the big game hunter Joseph DELMONT (1873–1937) had renounced hunting and had been filled with a loving attitude toward all creatures, he often stayed out all night in the jungle without a gun, quietly observing the beasts of prey without being harmed! Also the big-game hunt organizer in the Dutch East Indies, Johannes HOFER, lost overnight the desire to kill animals and then used to spend all day and night in the primeval forest conversing with the animals, and these were subject to the magic of his glance and of his voice. He often demonstrated in zoological gardens that he was able to pacify the rage of furious wild beasts by means of a few words whispered under his breath. "Worth remembering are the wild jungle creatures encountered by Sadhu SUNDAR SINGH (1889–1932) on his missionary journeys without being attacked by them or frightening them away."[408]

Dr. Hermann HAUPT (1922) is an advocate of HUTER'S system of spiritual healing who died in California in 1936. Haupt used to say of his preceptor: "HUTER often emphasized that love conquers all material things, and there is no disease that can permanently withstand the radiations of a loving will."[409]

Hans Heinrich EHRLER (1931), a one-time postal clerk and later Swabian poet (1872–1952) expressed the opinion: "I believe

---

[408]FRITSCHE, *Tierseele* [The Animal Psyche], p. 275; SCHRÖDTER: *Offenbarungen*, p. 61.
[409]HAUPT, p. 41.

a human being can be as full of love and kindness inside as to be able to cure disease." And he offered the following personal experience in proof of this: ". . . and, strange to say, my way led me to a fever-stricken young man, a student whose nerves had been shattered by the war. I stood at his bedside on my own and—*putting all my feelings into it*—I wished that the "fiery mantle" enveloping his poor body would dissolve. All at once two eyes looked up at me, and a mouth composed itself three times rather oddly to frame the following sentences separately: "Who are you? / Where have you come from? / It's doing me good!" With each sentence it was as if a wrapper was being taken off the sufferer. The agony left his face and he closed his eyes. The patient was well again.

Back home I knelt down and prayed that I might not presume to do anything that was beyond my legitimate scope. *Nevertheless, I truly believe that in one's lifetime one can be filled with so much love and kindness that one can heal the sick*, and that in the end we shall all be able to heal one another in body and mind."[410]

F. C. CARNACHON (1934), a researcher who talked with NYOKA, the Prince Imperial of the "Empire of the Snakes," a secret society in Tanganyika [modern Tanzania] was told that: "The 'snake men' are entrusted by *Limdini*—the great herdsman—with keeping his children safe and sound. To be a snake man one must above all have kind thoughts and pure truth in one's heart."[411]

Dr. Alexander HEERMANN (died 1946): This Paracelsian doctor, dowser, and former Surgeon-General was in possession of considerable authenticated *Psi-Gamma* abilities. The question of a friend—Dr. Ernst BUSSE (born 1893)—as to how he managed to perform such extraordinary cures, elicited the following reply: "They are possible only if one has a completely pure heart." That this was not arrogance and that this man, born in 1863, did have "pure truth in his heart," is shown by the following episode. One day when he was overtired and had fallen asleep before noon, he was wakened by a noisy exchange between his wife and a caller. His anxious wife was trying to get rid of the patient by pretend-

[410]EHRLER, H. Hch., *Briefe aus meinem Kloster* [Letters from My Cloister] (Lorch, 1931).
[411]CARNACHON, F. C. and ADAMSON, Hans Christian, *Das Kaiserreich der Schlangen* [The Empire of the Snakes] (Erlenbach bei Zürich, 1934), pp. 27–28; SCHRÖDTER, *Offenbarungen*, p. 76.

ing her husband was not at home. The doctor expostulated with his wife in the strongest possible terms, and asked her never again to make use of such falsehoods, *as otherwise he ran the risk of having his paranormal abilities taken away from him!*

In the fall of 1955, the USA medical world (and in 1957 the German public)[412] became aware of the work of Dr. John T. FERGUSON, who in 1954 was made Director of the Psychiatric Department in the Traverse City, MI hospital. The *Journal of the Medical Association of America* described the successful cures of mental disorders as "absolutely revolutionary" after the official Association of American Psychiatrists for the Middle West had spent a month supervising his trials on the "incurable." There are three things to say about FERGUSON, the not quite 50-year-old [at the time of writing] "father of the mad," and his mode of procedure. First, that he himself fell prey to a serious mental illness ("incurable" paranoia) due to overwork, disappointment, and narcotics. Second, his maxim: "Medicaments (narcotics) drove me insane; and medicaments can cure insanity!" This claim is not new; long ago the Atharva Veda of Ancient India recommended for insanity plants such as *Rauwolfia serpentina* (which has only now come to the attention of the West). FERGUSON treats his patients chiefly with a pill of his own preparation, which he has so far refused to name. His colleagues simply call them "Ferguson's pills." Third, the pill alone does nothing, it has to be taken. And something has to accompany it. FERGUSON'S wife Mary says: "John heals with chemistry and love!"

Johannes MÜLLER-ELMAU (1864–1949), was a theologian and writer. His fundamentally Christian attitude, although outside the pale of the Church, supported the worldly culture of the personality, and founded "sanctuaries of personal life" in Schloß Mainberg and later in Schloß Elmau, as well as publishing *Die Grünen Blätter* [Green Leaves]. He has presented us with a very beautiful leitmotiv that comes right to the point: "The vocation of a human being is to be the organ of God."

God is All-powerful + All-knowing + All-loving. But we must not try to emulate our Maker in the areas of power and

---

[412]BRANNER, Ralph T., "Ich heile Irrsinn mit Liebe" [I Cure Mental Derangement with Love], *7 Tage* (1957), 43 [Oct. 19]: 1, 4.

knowledge, but in spreading His love. For as PAUL, the prince of apostles, says: "Though I speak with the tongues of men and of angels, and have not charity, I am become as sounding brass, or a tinkling cymbal. And though I have the gift of prophecy, and understand all mysteries, and all knowledge; and though I have all faith, so that I could remove mountains, and have not charity, I am nothing. Charity never faileth: but whether there be prophecies, they shall fail; whether there be tongues, they shall cease; whether there be knowledge, it shall vanish away."[413]

And this is in order that they promise might be made good: *"I will bless thee . . . and thou shalt be a blessing!"* (Genesis 12:2).

---

[413] I Corinthians 13: 1, 2, 8.

INDEX
OF NAMES

APOLLONIUS	of Tyana. Neo-Pythagorean wonder-worker.	10–97 [?]	82
ARAM	Kurt; i.e., Hanns FISCHER. Author of travel books and learned historiographer of sorcery, magic, and mysticism.	1869–1934	11, 122
ATKINSON	William Walker. Attorney, "New Thought" writer; last years spent in Los Angeles.	1852–1932	40
AVICENNA	Abu Ali al-Hussein Ibn Sina. Celebrated Persian physician. His "Canon" was the standard medical work in the Middle Ages.	979–1036	27
BAAROVA	Lyda. Czech film actress, a favorite of GOEBBELS.	Contemporary	123
BACON	Roger. Franciscan in Oxford. Natural philosopher, alchemist, "Doctor mirabilis."	1214–1294	53
BAGNALL	Oscar. Englishman. Improved KILNER'S screens into "aura goggles."	Contemporary (1937)	96
BAKER-EDDY	Mary, née BAKER. North American lady, her third marriage was to sewing-machine representative A. G. EDDY. Founded "Christian Science" in 1866, and	1821–1910	109

published her *Science and
Health* in 1875.

BARBARIN	Georges. French popular philosopher.	Contemporary	59
BARKER	I. Ellis. English jounalist.	Born 1870	46
BARTOK	Eva. Hungarian film star, healed by *Subud*.	Born 1929	119
BASILIUS	Valentinus. Benedictine monk in St. Peter's monastery, Erfurt. Famous alchemist; hence his nickname "Magnus."	1413 Authenticated date.	102
BAUDOIN	Charles. Professor at the Institut J. J. Rousseau and lecturer on the Philosophy Faculty to Genevan COUÉ students.	Born 1893	74
BAVENT	Madeleine. Character in a novel by PRZYBYSZEWSKI.		80
BECHSTEIN	Johann Matthäus. Forester and ornithologist.	1757–1822	111
DI BELMONTE	Granito Pignatelli. Italian cardinal; alleged possessor of the "evil eye" (*jettatore*).	1851–1948	3
BÉNAMAR	Sidi Moulay Ali ben Lardi. Sheikh of the Ouled Sidi Bénamar family in	Contemporary	133, 134

Néromar (Algeria):
miracle healer.

BENDER	Hans, Ph.D., M.D. Professor, Director of the Inst. für Grenzgebiete der Psychologie und Psychohygiene, Freiburg i. Br., Germany.	Born 1907	24
BENEDIKT	Moritz, M.D. Professor of Neurology and Criminal Psychiatry at the University of Vienna; interested in dowsing problems.	1835–1920	13, 18
BENNETT	J. G. Introduced *Subud* to England; headquarters in Coombe Springs.	Contemporary	58, 62, 117, 118
BERGER	Hans, M.D. Professor at the University Nerve Clinic in Jena; starting in 1924, developed the *electroencephalograph.*	1873–1941	26
BERGSON	Henri, D. Litt. Foremost modern French philosopher, member of the "Académie française." "For him, intuition is the metaphysical organ of knowledge." Theory of *élan vital.*	1895–1941	25
BERNSTEIN	Lew. Researcher in Denver, CO.	Contemporary	141
BERTRAM	Karl. Keeper of public records, mesmerist in	Born 1878	49

Berlin-Steglitz.
"Mummification."
Distant healing.

Béziat	Jean. First of all a lecturer in agriculture, then a miracle healer on the "La Borrie" estate in Avignonet (Haute-Garonne).	Died 1927	130
Bier	August, M.D. Professor of Surgery in Berlin. Privy Councillor. National prize for science. "Beer congestion" (1903). Lumbar anesthesia. Electric knife.	1861–1949	10
Blavatsky	Helena Petrovna Blavatskaya (H.P.B.), née Hahn. Co-founder, in 1875, of The Theosophical Society.	1831–1891	144
Blesenius	Petrus; Pierre de Blois; Peter of Blois. Ended up as archdeacon in London.	1130–1212	viii
Blondlot	René-Prosper. Professor of physics in the University of Nancy; N(ancy)-rays (Charpentier).	1849–1930	21
Bloom	Leopold. Advertising agent in Dublin. Character in the novel Ulysses, by James Joyce.		5
Bloom	Molly. Singer in Dublin; wife of Leopold Bloom.		33

	Character in the novel, *Ulysses*, by James JOYCE.		
BLOSS	Wolff, M.D. G.P. in Bietigheim (Württ.). *Handflächenphänomen* [The Phenomenon of Palm Sensitivity] and the "cold mantle" detected at the reaction distance.	Contemporary	100
BÖSS	Julie, née KNIESE. Pendulum researcher in Weimar. Also wrote children's books. Husband a sculptor.	Contemporary	41
BOIRAC	Emile. French magistrate, philosopher, parapsychologist, residing in Dijon (Côte d'Or).	1851–1917	12
BOLTZIUS	Friedrich August. Swedish pastor; *Boltzianism*. Biomagnetic healing by wearing the clothing of a completely healthy person.	1836–1910	24
BONAPARTE	Joseph. Brother of NAPOLEON I. King of Naples (1806), of Spain (1808–1813); ailurophobe.	1768–1844	29
BOWLY	W. S., Dr. English psychologist (1953)	Contemporary	140
Boylan	Dublin citizen who was a character in JOYCE'S novel, *Ulysses*.		33

BRAVIAK	Hungarian man of learning. Demonstrated, by means of electrical apparatus, the so-called "life-field" in a dying man.	Contemporary (1949)	103
BROOK	Charles. English healer (former jurist). In 1953 gave successful spiritual treatment to the British Queen's racehorse "Aureole."	Contemporary	29
BROUARDEL	Prof. Paul Camille Hippolyte, M.D. Dean of the Medical Faculty, Paris.	1837–1906	126, 127
BRUNTON	Paul. Former London journalist, then follower of the *Maharishi*. Introduced Eastern philosophy to general public.	Born 1895	33, 145
BUDDHA	Originally, Gautama Siddharta. Indian prince, the "Buddha" ("enlightened"). Founder of *Buddhism*.	560–480 B.C.	142
BULWER	Edward George, Earl (Lord) LYTTON, Baron KNEBWORTH. English Secretary of State for the Colonies, novelist, practicing magician.	1803–1873	55
BUSSE	Ernst, M.D. Lay medical practitioner in Garmisch-Partenkirchen.	Born 1893	75, 146

Akupunkturfibel
[Acupuncture Primer]
(1954).

BUSSE	Hermann Eris. Author, saga-poet.	1891–1947	11
BUTTENSTEDT	Carl. Secretary of mines in Rüdersdorf bei Berlin. Brilliant private scholar (theory of flight, exchange of vital force), Honorary member of "La Stella d'Italia."	1845–1910	46
CAAN	Albert, M.D. First Assistant at the Institute for Cancer Research (1911), Heidelberg. Proved the radioactivity of human organs.	Contemporary	88
CALLEDO	M.D. G.P. in Noputo (Italy). Mesmerist.	ca. 1900	47
CARNACHON	F.C. African explorer from the USA.	Contemporary (1934)	146
CARREL	Alexis, M.D. French surgeon and pathologist, appointed professor at the Rockefeller Institute, NY, in 1909. Nobel prize 1912. "King of the tissue culturers" (explantation).	1873–1944	95
CARTESIUS	Renatus; René DESCARTES. French mathematician, physicist, astronomer, philosopher (Cartesianism). *Cogito ergo sum.*	1596–1650	32

CARUS	Carl Gustav, M.D. Professor. Physician to the royal house of Saxony, believer in vital magnetism, leading light of his age.	1781–1869	111
CARVER	George Washington. Black American, doctorate in chemistry. Chemist, philanthropist. Established own foundation.	1864–1943	137
CATO	the Elder, Marcus Portius. Austere Roman censor. Foe of Carthage (*Ceterum censeo*)	234–149 B.C.	72
CAZZAMALI	Ferdinando, M.D. Professor of Psychiatry at the University of Modena. Evidence of "brain rays." President of the Italian Scientific Association for Metaphysics.	Died 1958	26
Cellini	Rafaello. Young Italian painter. Character in CORELLI's novel, *A Romance of Two Worlds*.		50
CHARPENTIER	Pierre Marie Augustin, M.D. Professor of Physiology and Neurology at the University of Nancy. Assisted BLONDLOT in the discovery of "N-rays."	1852–1916	21
CHEVREUIL	Michel Eugène. French chemist.	1786–1889	40

	Chevreuil's Pendulum Experiments.		
CHVOSTEK	Franz, M.D. Viennese Internist. *Chvostek-Zeichen.*	1835–1884	4
COCKELL	Don. English light heavyweight boxer. In telepathic contact with MILLER during contests.	Born 1927	38
CODRINGTON	English missionary.	Contemporary	128
COEUR	Jacques. French Freemason Treasurer to King Charles VII of France.	1395–1456	90
COLD	Eberhard, Ph.D. Psychology of religion.	Contemporary (1940)	96
CORELLI	Marie. English novelist of Italian descent.	1864 [?]–1924	1, 4, 29, 50, 82
CORENTIN	Cécilie. French Tibetan explorer.	Contemporary (1937)	37
COTUGNO	also CUTONI, Dominico. Physician in ordinary to the King of Italy.	1736–1822	121
COUÉ	Emile. Pharmacist at Nancy; systematizer and popularizer of *Autosuggestion.*	1857–1926	65
CRILE	George Washington. University professor (biology) in Cleveland,	Born 1864	26

OH, photographed the radiations of human brain tissue.

DE CRINIS	Max. Professor at the Graz University Hospital; demonstrated the phosphorescence of brain tissue.	Born 1889	26, 73
CURRY	Manfred, M.D. Born in Boston, MA. Private researcher in Dießen (Ammersee). Bioclimatologist, "Aran," W(arm front) and C(old front) types. Today [i.e. at the time of writing] there is a Manfred Curry Clinic under the direction of HÄNSCHE.	1899–1953	98
DACQUÉ	Edgar. Munich paleontologist and philosopher.	1878–1945	32
DALI	Salvador. Surrealist, Spanish painter in USA.	Born 1904	32
DAUMER	Georg Friedrich. Schoolteacher in Nuremberg. Foster-father of Kaspar HAUSER; religious and philosophical author and poet.	1800–1875	19
DAVID-NEEL	Alexandra. French professor, expert on Tibet and Buddhism, "Lama-Dama" initiate ("Yellow Hat").	Born 1878	37, 112

DRIESCH	Hans. Biologist and philosopher; appointed professor in Leipzig in 1921. Founder of "neovitalism," which denies that organic processes are mechanical.	1867–1941	45
DURVILLE	Gaston, M.D. G.P. in Paris. Son of Hector DURVILLE.	Contemporary	48
DURVILLE	Hector. Professor at a private academy for biomagnetism. Photography of the human "fluid emanations" (ca. 1909).	1849–1923	88, 94
ECKEHART	Meister Eckehart [Eckhart]. Dominican; most influential Catholic mystic of the Middle Ages.	1260–1327	131
ECKERMANN	Johann Peter. Honorary doctor. GOETHE'S private secretary. *Goethe's Table Talk*.	1792–1854	81, 106
EHRLER	Hans Heinrich. Swabian poet.	1872–1952	145
EIGNER	Julius. Traveler in China and writer based in Münstermaifeld (1951).	Contemporary	81
EINTHOVEN	Willem. Dutch physiologist. Professor in Leiden. Nobel prize in 1924. Studied the action currents of the heart with	1860–1927	100

	the string galvanometer he invented.		
ENCAUSSE	See PAPUS.		
Evrard	Amy. Wife of an American officer in CORELLI'S novel, *A Romance of Two Worlds* (1886).		82
FERGUSON	John T. Appointed mental specialist in Traverse City Hospital (Michigan) in 1954. "Ferguson's pills."	Contemporary (1957)	147
VON FEUCHTERSLEBEN	Baron Ernst, M.D. Physician ("mental dietician") and philosopher based in Vienna.	1806–1849	5, 39, 85
FISCHER	Dr. Professor of Psychology at the University of Marburg a. d. L. Studied (1949) GRÖNING in Herford	Contemporary	47
FISCHER	Oskar. Professor of Psychiatry in the University of Prague. Expert witness in the HANUSSEN case in 1929.	Contemporary	25
FISHER	Betty, M.D. G.P. in Philadelphia, PA. Advocate of "silence therapy." (1955)	Contemporary	139
FLASSER	Artur. Graduated engineer in München-Obermenzing.	Born 1886	114
FRIEDRICH II	Staufenkaiser.	1215–1250	140

FRITSCHE	Herbert, Ph.D. Biology, Metabiology. Noted, among other things, for his work on Homeopathy. Lived in Munich.	Born 1911	29
GALTON	Sir Francis. English traveler and scientist. Anticipated Chevreuil's pendulum research.	1822–1911	40
GATES	Elmer. Professor of Psychology in the "Pennsylvania School of Industrial Art." New-type psychological experiments in the psychology laboratory of the University of Washington in 1879; hence *Psychurg!*	1859–1923	85
GEMASSMER	Josef, M.D. G.P. in Berlin-Grunewald, first president of the "Society for the Promotion of Spiritual Healing" (at that place). "Meditative ecstasy" of the healer, and "meditative resonance of the patient" through the transfer of "regenerating impulses."	Contemporary	46, 54, 55, 56, 58
GEORGE	Stefan (Etienne). Lyric poet and translator. Verse was strictly formal and sometimes mannered.	1868–1933	105, 106
GICHTEL	Johann Georg. Originally an attorney. Visionary and mystic. *Gichtelaner* or *Engelbrüder* still exist in North	1638–1710	102

	Germany and The Netherlands. *Theosophia Practica* (1701–1708).		
GOEBBELS	Paul Joseph. Minister of the Reich for Public Enlightenment and Propaganda. Patron of BAAROVA.	1897–1945	123
VON GOETHE	Johann Wolfgang. Famous author.	1749–1832	3, 6, 33, 34, 68, 81, 106, 114, 143
GRATZINGER	Josef, M.D. G.P. in Vienna. Mesmerist.	Died 1924	13, 15, 19
GRAUPNER	Heinz, M.D. Noted medical writer in Munich.	Born 1906	140
DE GRIGNAN	Françoise Marguerite. Countess. Daughter of the Marquise DE SÉVIGNÉ, intelligent, polyglot: la plus jolie fille de France [the prettiest girl in France].	1646–1705	72
GRÖNING	i.e. GRÖNKOWSKY, Bruno. Naturally gifted; discovered his own suggestion method; possessed definite magnetic powers. Lived in Plochingen/Neckar.	1906–1959	23, 47

GROGGER	Paula. Styria. Author inspired by her native land.	Born 1892	91
GRUBER	Karl, M.D. Assistant professor of biology and zoology at the Technical College in Munich. Parapsychological studies.	1881–1927	55
GRUNEWALD	Fritz. Engineer in Berlin-Charlottenburg. "Physical Mediumism Researches" (1920).	Died 1925	21, 101
GÜNDL	Käthe. Honorary Ph.D. from the private Université Philotechnique (Brussels). Former health practitoner ("G-waves"—radar diagnosis). Radiation researcher and author in Vienna.	Born 1881	75, 76
GUYON	Jeanne Marie Bouvières de la Mothe G. French quietist mystic.	1648–1717	33
HÄNIG	Hans. Retired assistant teacher in Leipzig. Parapsychological publications.	Contemporary	101
HÄNSCHE	Hans Adolf, M.D. Chief physician of the Manfred Curry Clinic in Riederau (Ammersee). The human electrical field.	Contemporary	66, 97, 98
HAGERTY	James C. Press Officer to [President] Dwight David Eisenhower.	Contemporary	60

HAIDER	Maria. Austrian. Experienced so-called "shared sensations."	Contemporary (1958)	53
VON HALLER	Albrecht. Swiss anatomist, physiologist, botanist, and poet. Professor in Göttingen. "Haller's acid" (a mixture of sulf. acids).	1708–1777	115
HANUSSEN	Erik Jan; properly HERSCHMANN STEINSCHNEIDER. Telepath and clairvoyant, whose "mysterious spiritual powers" were certified in the "Leitmeritz clair-voyant case" in 1929. *My Life Line* (1930).	1889–1933	25
VON HARTMANN	Eduard. Philosopher. *Philosophie des Unbewußten* [Philosophy of the Unconscious] (1869).	1842–1906	77
HARTMANN	Franz, M.D. G.P. in the USA. On his return to Germany, initiated the "Lignosulfitheilweise" [Lignosulphite therapy]. Leader of the German "Lotusblüten" [Lotus Flower] Theosophists.	1838–1912	10, 39, 40, 50, 51, 76, 78, 136
HASEGAWA	Hiro. Japanese American. Ju-Jitsu instructor in the Police Academies of the State of California, and later in Chicago.	Contemporary	107

HAUFFE	Christina Friederica, née Wanner. Somnambulist (trance subject). *The Seeress of Prevorst* (Kreis Gronau in Württemberg). Observed and described by KERNER, then district physician in Weinsberg bei Heilbronn.	1801–1829	47
HAUPT	Hermann, LL.D. Follower of HUTER.	Died 1936	145
HAUSER	Kaspar. Foundling: Nuremberg, 1828. Mystery surrounds his origins: crown prince of Baden? Stabbed to death in 1833 (by Major VON HENNEBERG?). At the time of writing 3000 books had been published about him.	1812[?]–1833	5, 47
HEERMANN	Alexander, M.D. G.P. in Cassel. Surgeon-General retired. Researched dowsing and radiation, anticipated penicillin.	1863–1946	20, 49, 146
HEIM	Albert. Swiss geologist and Alpine explorer.	1849–1937	43
HEIM	Ernst Ludwig, M.D. Popular G.P. in Berlin. "Old Heim."	1747–1834	5
HEIN	Egon M. Engineer and currently [at the time of writing] only certified magnetizer in	Born 1893	116, 117

telegraphy with NETHERCOT
in 1949. Lived in
Evanston, IL.

IMMERMANN	Karl Leberecht. Senior provincial court official, stage-manager and poet in Düsseldorf.	1796–1840	5, 124
IRANSCHÄR	Hossein Kazemzadeh. Doctor's son from Tabriz (Iran), "Licencié en sciences pol. et sociales" [B.Sc. in social and political science], public lecturer in philosophy in Deggersheim (Canton of St. Gallen) since 1936. Founded an esoteric school there in 1942.	Born 1884	139
ISENBERG	Carl D., M.D. Hamburg G.P. Saw many functional psychoses as possession phenomena.	1876–1941	136
ISRAEL	Ben Elieser. Baal Shem Tov (= "Master of the Good Name," i.e., of God), commonly known as the Besht. Founder of Chasidism. Kabbalist and thaumaturge.	1700–1760	77, 81
IVERSEN	Dorothea. The "miracle-worker" of Copenhagen Taubenweg possessed powerful healing magnetism. Also performed distant healing over the phone.	Born 1899	19
JAEGER	Gustav, M.D. Professor of Zoology, hygienist ("wool	1832–1917	31, 110

regime"). G.P. in Stuttgart.
Believed in mental emana-
tions and biomagnetism.

Janus	Meister Janus. Character in *Axel*, posthumous work of VILLIERS DE L'ISLE ADAM.		117
JESUS CHRIST		7 B.C.–A.D. 26	135, 136, 138, 140
JOHANNSEN	Peter. Danish medium, magnetizer, lived in Copenhagen. GRUNEWALD'S test subject. 1917–1920.	Contemporary	21
JOHN	John the Baptist (Yochanan the Immerser) Essene-type baptizer and ascetic. "Metanoeite!" [Repent!] Christian era.		135
JOHN	The beloved disciple. Evangelist.	Died A.D.? 100	145
JOYCE	James. Irish author, whose *Ulysses* has had a prodigious influence on modern literature. It is the psychoanalytically viewed 24-hour "odyssey" of an average man.	1882–1941	5, 33, 39, 84
JUDAH BEN JACOB	Son of the patriarch *Jacob* (Ya'akov). Pledged his divining rod and divining ring to his (unrecognized) daughter-in-law THAMAR as security	1800 B.C.	42

for payment for an hour
of love (Genesis ch. 38).

JÜRGENS	Heinrich. Medical pedagogue. Mesmerist. "The Vedantist from the Hotzenwalde" (but actually came from Cologne).	Contemporary	139
JUNG	Carl Gustav. Swiss psychoanalyst. Mental specialist and philosopher. The "collective unconscious"; "archetypes."	Born 1875	77
JUNG-STILLING	Heinrich Jung, surnamed "Stilling." Originally a tailor, then a doctor. The most famous cataract operator in Goethe's time. Finally Professor of Political Economy in Heidelberg. Mystic, author.	1740–1817	102
KAGAWA	Toyochiko, Dr. theol. Independent Christian evangelist in Japan.	Born 1888	132
KARL I	Karl der Große, Carolus Magnus, Charlemagne. King of France. Holy Roman Emperor in 800.	768–814	32
KARL VII	Charles VII of France, the "victorious." Sovereign of COEUR and of the "Maid of Orléans," JOAN OF ARC.	1422–1461	90

KERNER	Andreas Justinus Christian, M.D. Head physician in Weinsberg bei Heilbronn. *Seeress of Prevorst* (1829). His *Klecksographie* [Ink-blotography] uses the Rohrschach Test.	1786–1862	128
KERNING	J.B.; real name Joh. Bapt. KREBS. Reviver of the so-called "alphabet letter exercises" ("Kerning mysticism") in which letters imagined on the skin are supposed to lead to the "inner word."	1774–1849	91
KILNER	Walter J. Attached to St. Thomas's Hospital in London. Invented "Kilner screens" which allegedly enable non-sensitives to see the aura.	Contemporary	36, 96
KINDBORG	Erich, M.D. G.P. in Breslau (1922).	Contemporary	12
KLUGE	Carl Alexander Ferdinand, M.D. Professor of surgery in the Royal Prussian Military Academy. One of the most celebrated mesmerists of his period.	1782–1844	36, 121
KORSCHELT	Oskar. Instructor in Chemistry at the Imperial University of Tokyo 1876–1884. Later on in Dresden invented the	1841–1939[?]	94

	so-called "solar ether radiation apparatus."		
KRAFT	Robert. Sailor and popular writer of fantastic tales. "Trance writer."	1869–1916	38
KRAMER	Philipp Walburg. Past master of German magnetizers with quite considerable, even medically certified success. *In extremis* recommended "collective magnetizing" by several healthy operators working in unison.	1815–1899	19
KRÖNER	Walter, M.D. G.P. in Berlin. Well-known parapsychological writer.	Contemporary	8
KUNGEYUAK	Aged Eskimo on the east coast of Greenland. Rescued North Americans who had made an emergency landing.	Contemporary (1955)	129
LACOMBE	Pater. Madame GUYON's confessor.	ca. 1700	33
LAFONTAINE	Charles. One of the most eminent mesmerists of his era.	Ca. 1860	3, 14, 42
LAKHOVSKY	Georges. Professor in Paris. *Cosmic Rays and Vital Vibrations* (1931).	Contemporary	7
LALANDE	Emanuel Henri; M.D.; alias MARC HAVEN. G.P. in Lyons. Son-in-law of "MAÎTRE PHILIPPE."	1868–1926	126, 127

LANGBEIN	H., (M.D.?) in Niederlößnitz (Sa.). Attributed the path of the pendulum to radioactivity of the human body. (CAAN).	Contemporary (1914)	88
LAO TSZE	Properly LI-PEK-YANG. Archivist at the court of TSCHÉU. Founder of Taoism.	604–514 [?]	138
LASKY	Ludwig, M.D. Medical specialist in Vienna. Mesmerist, trained by GRATZINGER.	Contemporary (1922)	13, 15
LASSALLE	Ferdinand; properly LASAL. Jurist, writer, socialist leader; fell in duel for Helene v. DÖNNIGES-RACOWITZA.	1825–1864	50
LAWRENCE	Brother (Nicholas HERMAN). French Carmelite.	1610–1691	136
LEAVITT	Sheldon, M.D. Professor in the Gynecological Institute Chicago. New Thought physician and writer. *Paths to the Heights* (1908).	1848–1933	61
LEE	Frederick George. Blood donor and porter at Middlesex Hospital in England.	Born 1901	70
LEGRAND	Teddy. Parisian writer.	Contemporary (1936)	81

LEISBERGER	M.D. Austrian brain scientist.	Contemporary	67, 68
LERMINA	Jules. French journalist and author.	Died 1915	116
LEWANEVSKY	Sigismund. Russian polar aviator. Search and rescue attempt by WILKINS (1937).	Contemporary	37
LÉVY-BRUHL	Lucien. D.Litt. French professor of philosophy. Studies on the mode of thought of [so-called] primitive races.	1857–1938	52
LHOTZKY	Heinrich. German clergyman and author in Southern Russia.	1859–1930	71, 80
LIEK	Erwin, M.D. G.P. and writer. *Das Wunder in der Heilkunde* [Miracle in Medicine].	1878–1935	62
LORCA	Federico Garcia. Spanish poet.	1899–1936	138
LÜ BÜ WE	Chinese Chancellor under TSIN SHI HUANG DI (246–210 B.C.). Patron of arts and letters. *The Spring and Fall of Lü-Bü-We.*	Died 232 B.C.	69
LUTZE	Arthur M.D. Member of the Board of Health in Cöthen i.A. One of the first and first-rate Homeopaths among doctors.	1803–1870	87, 143
MAETERLINCK	Maurice Polydore Marie Bernard. Belgian	1862–1949	30

	playwright, lyric poet, essayist, scientist, non-fiction books. Nobel prize 1911.		
MARAIS	Eugène Nielen. South African. Termite research worker.	Died 1937	30
Margarethe	Character in GOETHE'S *Faust*.		3
MARK	Evangelist.	Died A.D. [?] 80	140
MATTHIAS	Eugen. Private researcher in Zürich. Professor of Biophysics 1924–1937. Mechano-therapy in Munich. "Matthias-aggregate."	1882–1958	112, 113, 114, 138
McDOUGALL	William. Animal psychologist at Duke University, Durham, NC. Assistant to RHINE from 1930.	1875–1938	24
Mephistopheles	Character in GOETHE'S *Faust. Megist-ophi-les* (Greek: "Great serpent spirit"), or *Mustafil* (Arabic: "one who performs something").		3
MESMER	Franz Anton, M.D. Rediscoverer of healing magnetism; named for him—"Mesmerism."	1733–1815	55
MEYER	Conrad Ferdinand. Swiss narrative writer and lyric poet. (Mentally deranged from 1891).	1825–1898	35

MEYRINK	Gustav. Occult writer, practicing yogi.	1868–1932	9, 10, 17, 120, 124
MICHAEL	Gert, D. Psychol. Columnist for *Heim und Welt* (Hanover).	Contemporary	139
MILLER	S.W.J. Psychotherapist in Earsfield (England) in telepathic contact with COCKELL.	Contemporary (1949)	38
MLAKER	Rudolf. Retired colonel in Vienna. Researcher into pendulum dowsing. *Mental dowsing* (of the "chakras").	Born 1899	102
MOINEAU	M.D. French doctor, invented apparatus for measuring the electromagnetic waves in humans.	Contemporary (1930)	100
MORGENSTERN	Christian. Poet, philosopher, anthroposophist.	1871–1914	40
DE MOROGIAFFERI	Parisian top attorney, defender of ALALOUF.	1872–1956 [?]	134
MOSES	Egyptian: *Osarsiph.* Israelite adopted by Egyptian princess THERMUTIS [?]. Instructed in "all the wisdom of the Egyptians" [perhaps] in the temple university, Heliopolis.	1225 B.C.	89

MOUTIN	Lucien, M.D. French G.P. Discovered the "Moutin reflex" for estimating the suggestibility of a test subject.	1856–1919	19
MÜLLER	E.K. Electronic engineer in Kilchberg-Zürich. Director of the "Salus." Discoverer, *Anthropoflux*.	1853–1948	20, 43, 88, 89
MÜLLER-CZERNY	Gustav Adolf (Egmont Roderich). "The miracle doctor of Homburg." Spiritual healer in the style of GRÖNING. Philanthropist.	1862–1922	130
MÜLLER-ELMAU	Johannes. Theologian and writer. "Sanctuaries of personal life" at Schloß Mainau, Schloß Elmau.	1864–1949	147
MÜLLER-GUTTENBRUNN	Herbert, Ph.D. Publisher and editor of the monthly review of current affairs *Das Nebelhorn*.	Died 1945	8
MUJAGITSCH	Mustapha Efendi. Retired auditor. Moslem. Miracle healer of Sarajevo. Healed specific snake bites, even over the telephone!	Born 1875	132, 134
NAPOLEON	Bonaparte. Emperor of France 1804–1814 (1815).	1769–1821	29, 119
VON NARKIEWICZ-JODKO	Jakob. Russian privy counsellor and scientist. Member of the "Imperial	Turn of the century	96

Institute for Century
Experimental Medicine"
in St. Petersburg.
Elektrographie of the hand
rays.

NETHERCOT	A. M. Dr. in Northwestern University (USA). Reported in 1949 to have invented infra-red tele-graphy with HUXFORD.	Contemporary (1949)	99
NETTESHEIM	Heinrich Cornelius Agrippa von Nettesheim bei Trier. Imperial knight, captain, and councilor. "Imperator" of a "sodality" (society for scientific and psychic research). Was in tele-pathic communication with his teacher, the "wizard abbot" TRITHEMIUS. (*Occult Philosophy*, Bk. I, ch. 6).	1486–1535	1, 34, 53, 110, 115
NEWTON	Dr. "Most celebrated American clairvoyant healing medium" (Dr. Gg. v. LANGSDORF). Cured Dr. Franz HARTMANN from a distance in the USA.	Died 1895	76
NICOLSON	Ph.D. Healer in Ragusa (Dubrovnik). The ideal example of a doctor in *Surya's Mod. Rosenkreuzer* [Modern Rosicrucians] (1907, 1930).		107

NIETZSCHE	Friedrich Wilhelm. Professor of Classical Philosophy in Basel. Philosopher (Superman, master morality, "will to power," eternal return, "transvaluation of all values"). Mentally ill after 1889. (Yajé-abuse?)	1844–1900	ix
NÜSSLEIN	Heinrich. Trance painter of Nuremberg; almost blind, created the "picture-writer" and thousands of "color prayers"; mummified with his hands.	1879–1947	48
VON NUSSBAUM	Johann Nepomuk, M.D. Royal Bavarian clinician and surgeon. G.P., Privy Councilor, professor of medicine. Recognized animal magnetism.	1829–1890	15, 83
NYOKA	Crown prince of a secret society of "snake men" among the natives of Tanzania (CARNACHON). (1934)	Contemporary	146
OCKEL	Gerhard, M.D. G.P. in Guben.	Contemporary (1936)	61
OSIANDER	Johann Friedrich, M.D. Professor at the University of Göttingen. Royal Waldeck Hofrat.	1787–1855	141
OSTY	Eugène, M.D. G.P. Parapsychologist. Director of the "Institut Métapsychique" in Paris.	1874–1938	2

PAPUS	I.E. Gérard Anaclet VINCENT ENCAUSSE, M.D. G.P., gynecologist in Paris, surgeon-colonel in World War I. Martinist leader. Practicing magician. With PHILIPPE at the court of the Czar.	1865–1926	70, 126, 127
PARACELSUS	Philippus Aureolus Theophrastus. Styled: Bombastus P. von Hohenheim. *Lutherus Medicorum* [The Luther of Physicians], the "King of doctors" in Renaissance times.	1493–1541	18, 58, 85, 110, 115, 127, 130, 143
Paris	Prince of Troy. By the rape of Helen ignited the Trojan war [in Homer's *Iliad*]. Makes an appearance in GOETHE'S *Faust*.		6
PATANJALI	Compiler of Raja Yoga sutras.	A.D. 200	79, 95
PAUL	Hebrew name: SAUL. Tent-maker, rabbin. Some while after his Damascus road experience, he became known as Paul. Apostle to the Gentiles.	Died A.D. 62 [?]	104, 127, 135, 136, 138, 148
PETER	Simon bar Jona. Fisherman on the Sea of Galilee. Apostle to the Jews.	Died A.D. [?] 64	104
PÉTETIN	Jacques Henri Désiré. Mesmerist of Lyons. In	1744–1808	20

	1805 explained "animal magnetism" in terms of "animal electricity."		
PEYREFITTE	Roger. Attaché to the French Embassy in Rome. Well-informed writer on political affairs.	Contemporary (1956)	3
VON PFAUNDLER	Professor (M.D.) Leading pediatrician. Reaction to *B. coli* and *Proteus* named for him.	Born 1879	140
PFEIFFER	Ehrenfried, M.D. Anthroposophic researcher. *Crystal image diagnosis* (1936). Lived at Threefold Farm, Spring Valley, NY.	Born 1899	88
PHILIPPE	Nizier Anthèlme. Thaumaturge of Lyons. The *Maître spirituel* of PAPUS, who presented him at the court of the Czar. Russian army surgeon with the rank of major-general. LALANDE'S father-in-law.	1849–1905	126, 127, 128
PICASSO	Pablo. Spanish painter based in France. Controversial paintings, graphics, and ceramics.	Born 1881	39
PIDDINGTON	Australian husband and wife. Put on a very convincing telepathic performance for BBC radio in London.	Contemporary (1949)	37

PITZER	Franz Xaver. Former Chief Constable of Munich.	Contemporary (1949)	47
POULSEN	Erling. Danish poet. His book *Notlandung* [Emergency Landing] was awarded a prize by the Scandinavian Society of Authors.	Contemporary (1956)	129
DU PREL	Baron Carl, Ph.D. Scholarly Bavarian occultist and spiritist. Classic author in the border sciences.	1839–1899	47
PRZYBYSZEWSKI	Stanislav. Polish writer. Satanist mystic.	1868–1927	80
PUYSÉGUR	Armand Marie Jacques de Chastenet, Marquis de Puységur. Noted mesmerist.	1751–1825	143
VON PYCHLAU	E. St. Petersburg learned man and Privy Counselor. Friend of E. K. MÜLLER.	Contemporary (1912)	43
PYTHAGORAS	Philosopher of Samos, music theorist, mathematician ("Pythagoras' theorem"). Founder of the "Pytha-gorean Brotherhood." Number speculation and mysticism ("Mathesis"). *Golden Verses.*	580–493 B.C.	87
RAMANA	Sri Ramana Maharishi ("Great Sage"). The "Bhagavan" of Tiruvan-namalai (South India).	1879–1950	81

	Indian holy man (BRUNTOIN, FRITSCHE, SCATCHERD, VON VELTHEIM-OSTRAU, ZIMMER).		
RAM DAS	Indian Swami [Hindu religious teacher].	Contemporary	ix
REEH	Johann-Jost. Physicist (graduated engineer) in Bad Ems, constructed with SCHWAMM a piece of apparatus for measuring the infrared radiation of humans.	Born 1927	98
REGAZZONI	Antonio. Mesmerist-cum-magician from Bergamo (upper Italy). Given a big build-up by SCHOPENHAUER. Made a sensationally successful tour of Europe in 1859. His speciality was *Foudroiement à distance*, or blasting a person to the ground from a distance, as if with a bolt of lightning.	Died 1870	130
REHDER	Hans, M.D. Medical superintendent of a clinic for gastric disorders in Hamburg-Altona. (1955).	Contemporary	65
VON REICHENBACH	Baron Karl. Scientist and industrialist with doctorate, living in Vienna. Discoverer of creosote, paraffin, and "Od" (1850).	1788–1869	12, 19, 21, 112
REIL	Johann Christian, M.D. Director of the hospitals in Halle/Saale. Fever	1759–1813	115

theory. "Reil lines,"
"Reil finger."

RETING	Hutuktu. Gyalpo or regent in Lhasa until November 16, 1950.	Contemporary (1950)	96
RHINE	Joseph Banks, Ph.D. Founder of "Parapsy-chological laboratory" (1930) at Duke University in Durham, NC, where he was professor. "E(xtra) S(ensory) P(erception)."	Born 1895	ix, 24, 26
RIECKE	G.P. in Stuttgart; mesmerist.	ca. 1819	129
RIEDLIN	Gustav, M.D. and Dr. of Naturopathy. Doyen of German doctors, advocating fasting; medical reformer, parapsychologist.	1862–1949	92
DE RIENCOURT	Amaury. French Tibetologist. *Tibet im Wandel Asiens* [Tibet in the Changes Facing Asia].	Contemporary (1956)	37
VAN RIJNBERK	Gérard A., M.D. Professor of Physiology in the University of Amsterdam. Parapsychological author.	1875–1953	82, 96, 104, 126
RILLSTROEM	Putative professor at the University of Uppsala, who was said to have measured the "sympathy radiation" between people (before 1952).	Contemporary (1950 [?])	71, 142

RINGGER	Peter, Ph.D. Parapsychologist in Oberengstringen bei Zürich; President of the "Swiss Para-Psychological Society." Author of *Neue Wissenschaft* [New Science], and *Das Weltbild der Parapsychologie* [The World-Picture of Parapsychology] (1959).	Born 1923	36
ROHLFS	Dora, M.D. G.P. in Munich. Affirmed the existence of human "biological force fields" able to survive death.	Born 1892	103
ROSENCREUTZ	A. Christian; Latin: *Rosicrucius*. Reputed renovator of the natural and spiritual sciences. Hidden Order of the *Rosicrucians* (*Fratres Roseae Crucis* [Brethren of the Rosy Cross]).	1378–1484	76, 131
RÜCKERT	Friedrich. Lyric poet. Imitator of highly formal Oriental poetry.	1788–1866	144
RUEFF	Jakob. Distinguished German gynecologist of some centuries ago.	ca. 1554	141
DE SAINT-MARTIN	Louis Claude. "The unknown philosopher." Mystical French philosopher. Illuminatist. Votary of Jakob BÖHME (1575–1624).	1743–1803	82

DE SAN ROMAN	Francisco di Borja. Spanish doctor who used the pendulum to make "aura diagnoses."	Contemporary (1956)	106
SANT MOTA	Venerated clairvoyant Hindu who was about 60 years old when visited by RAMDAS.	Turn of century	ix
SCHÄFER	Ernst. Indian-Tibetan expedition 1938/1939. *"The festival of the white veils"* made into the film "Geheimes Tibet."	Born 1911	96
SCHALECK	Robert, LL.D. President of the Superior District Court in the "Leitmeritz clairvoyant" action against HANUSSEN.	Contemporary	25
VON SCHILLER	Johann Christoph Friedrich.	1759–1805	86
SCHLAFFHORST-ANDERSEN	Leader of an innovative school of singing and breath-control in Heide bei Celle.	Contemporary (1934)	41
SCHLEICH	Karl Ludwig, M.D. Privy Councilor, professor of surgery, author and poet in Berlin.	1859–1922	30, 100, 120
SCHOPENHAUER	Arthur, Ph.D. Philosopher. The World as Will and Representation (1819). Adherent of mesmerism.	1788–1860	15, 138

Schultz	Johannes Heinrich, M.D. Professor and mental specialist in Berlin-Charlottenburg. Creator of "Autogenic Training" (1934).	1884–1970	41, 57
Schwab	Sophie. Wife of the mythologist Gustav Schwab (1792–1850).	Ca. 1830	128
Schwamm	Ernst, M.D. G.P. in Obernhof (Lahn). Psychosomatic therapy. Constructed with Reeh a piece of equipment for measuring infrared radiations in humans (early diagnosis!).	Born 1912	98
"Schwarzbart"	["Blackbeard"]. Chinese hermit in the Huang-Chan mountains.	Contemporary (1951)	81
Von Sebottendorf	Baron Rudolf. Adopted engineer Glauer. Astrologer. Published the psychic training of the Bektashi Dervishes.	1875–1935 [?]	75
Sédir	Paul; i.e. Yvon Leloup. French occultist, but since 1919 exclusively a mystic. Evangelic esotericist, pupil of "Maître Philippe."	1871–1926	54, 120
Seidl	Johann Gabriel. Treasurer of the Household and poet in Vienna. Wrote the second version of Haydn's	1804–1875	35

"Kaiser-Hymne" ("God keep, God save, our Emperor and our land!").

Sellin	Wilhelm Alfred. Retired colonial governor in Munich. Mesmerist. Friend of Thetter.	1841–1933	94
Severn	Arthur. English landscape painter, formed a "unit of emotion and sensation" with his wife.	Contemporary	50, 90
De Sévigné	Marie de Rabutin-Chantal, Marquise. French author.	1626–1696	72
Sherman	American author. Maintained telepathic contact with Wilkins in 1937.	Contemporary (1937)	37
De Silva	Richard, M.D. Attached to the Institute for Medical Research in Ceylon [now Sri Lanka]. Tested the possible influence of thought on bacterial growth.	Contemporary (1953)	53
Sommer	M.D. Psychotherapist in Stuttgart.	Contemporary (1958)	66
Spitz	René, M.D. Child psychiatrist. The "Spitz effect."	Born 1887	141
Stekel	Wilhelm, M.D. G.P. in Vienna. Dream researcher.	Born 1868	40

STERNEDER	Hans. Austrian author in Bregenz.	Born 1889	34, 83, 120
STEWART	I., M.D. Physician in the University Hospital in Bristol, England.	Contemporary (1950)	59
STIEFVATER	Erich W., M.D. G.P. in Freiburg/Br. Brilliant promoter of acupuncture and its philosophy.	Contemporary	x
STIFTER	Adalbert. Inspector of schools. Classic Sudeten German writer.	1805–1868	56
STRINDBERG	August. Swedish playwright. Student of medicine. Acute observer of background influences. Friend of SHLEICH.	1868–1912	5, 27, 112, 120
STRÖMBERG	Gustav. Professor. Director of the Mount Wilson Solar Observatory in Pasadena, CA. Demonstrated the (electrical) "Life Fields" in humans.	Born 1882	102, 103
SUBUH	Muhammad. Styled "Pak" (Little Father). At one time in government service in Middle Java. Founder of the *Subuh* spiritual awakening movement, which (as a by-product) is reported to have healing effects.	Born 1901	117

VON SUCHTEN	Alexander. Parcelsist. Alchemist.	Ca. 1550	124
SUNDAR SINGH	The *Sadhu* (Sanskrit: "holy man"). Practised Christian mysticism, chiefly in Tibet.	1899–1932	145
SURYA	G. W. *Surya* (Indian: "Sun," "Solar man"; Latin: *Solarius*). G. W. = GEORGIEWICZ-WEITZER; first name: Demeter. Austrian mechanical engineer. For many years the editor of the *Zentralblatt für Okkultismus* [Central News-sheet for Occultism] (Leipzig). Private scholar, finally living in Salzburg. Restorer of *Occult Medicine* (compilation).	1873–1949	50, 75, 107, 109, 134, 142, 144
SUSANNE	"Naughty Susanne." Barmaid in Los Angeles (CA).	1950	81
T.	M. T. Factory manager's wife in telepathic contact with her sleeping children, as reported by GRUBER.	Contemporary (1926)	55
TABRIZI	Hadji Ahmad al T. Dervish in Kerind (Northern Persia). Visited by BENNETT in 1955.	Born ca. 1880	134
TAWARA	Sunao. Japanese pathologist and anatomist in the Imperial Kynshu University. Discovered the	Born 1873	92

	Tawara nodes in the human heart, also the *Aschoff-Tawara nodes*, also named for the pathologist Dr. Ludw. ASCHOFF (1866–1942) in Freiburg/Br.		
TELLMANN	Professor. Russian scientist who found asylum in the [former] West German Republic.	1951	77
TENHAEFF	Wilhelm H.C. Leading Dutch parapsy-chologist, installed in 1953 as first professor of the newly established Department of Parapsy-chology at the University of Utrecht and as director of its Parapsychological Institute.	Born 1894	56
TENZEL	Andreas. "Philosopher and former Schwarzburg physician in ordinary," the "Gustav Jaeger of the XVIIth century" (KIESEWETTER), known for his *Medicina diastatica* or "In die Ferne würkende Arzneykunst" [Remote-acting therapy] of Anno 1629.	ca. 1600	46
TERSTEGEN	Gerhard. Silk ribbon worker in Mülheim, mystic, religious (Reformed) song writer, pietistical preacher.	1697–1769	136

THADDÄUS	Thaddée. Pseudonym of a miracle-worker in Paris ("Le Guérisseur de Plaisance") [The Healer of Plaisance].	1936	81
THAMAR	Widow of ER, son of the patriarch JACOB, with whom she lay after disguising herself (Genesis ch. 38).	2000 B.C.	42
THEODERICH	The Great. Ostrogoth king. *Dietrich von Bern* (Verona) of the Germans, *Thidrek* of the Northern Saga. MÜLLER-CZERNY regarded him as his spiritual helper.	471–526	130
THERMUTIS	Egyptian princess, daughter of Pharaoh MENEPHTAH. Mother [by adoption] of MOSHE (Moses)[?]. Her name reveals that she was a high-degree initiate.	1225 B.C.	89
THETTER	Rudolf. Engineer, later magnetizer in Vienna; the only approved pupil of GRATZINGER.	1882–1957	17, 18, 22
THOLUCK	August, D.D. Professor of Evangelical Theology in Halle/Saale.	1799–1877	5, 19
TISCHNER	Rudolf, M.D. Practiced in Icking bei Münich. Initially an ophthalmologist.	Born 1879	43

Historian and methodologist of Homeopathy. Nestor [wise old man] of German parapsychological research and one very well versed in its history.

TORMIN	Ludwig. Well-known magnetizer. Son-in-law of the famous vital-force healer KRAMER.	Turn of the century.	115
TRAMPLER	Kurt, LL.D. Remote healer in München-Gräfeling. Writer. *Lebenserneuerung durch den Geist.* [Life Renewal Through the Spirit].	Born 1904	23
TRINE	Ralph Waldo. Optimist. Popular philosopher in USA. *In Tune with the Infinite* (1905).	1866–1958	x, 52
TRITHEMIUS	Johannes. Real name HEIDENBERG of Trittenheim/Mosel. Abbot in Spanheim bei Kreuznach, then at St. Jakob in Würzburg-Vorstadt. Engaged in esoteric research; kept in telepathic contact with AGRIPPA.	1462–1516	102
TROMP	S.W., Dr. Geological adviser to the UN, parapsychologist in The Netherlands. *Psychical Physics* (1949).	Contemporary	100

Tsagalos	Ari, M.D. G.P. in Greece.	Contemporary (1955)	139
Tsin Schi Huang-Di	First Emperor of the Chinese Tsin dynasty. Forged the Chinese Empire, the "Yellow Napoleon."	246–210 B.C.	69
Tucci	Giuseppe. Italian professor and Tibetologist. Convert to Buddhism.	Contemporary	37
Von Tucher	Baron Gottlieb. District Assembly member, guardian of Kaspar Hauser.	ca. 1828	5, 19
Tuzlo	Shakir. *Hadji* (pilgrim to Mecca), *Hafiz* (Muslim who knows the Koran by heart), *Effendi* (educated man) in Sarajevo. Teacher of Mujagitsch.	Died 1944	133
Twain	Mark. Real name Samuel Langhorne Clemens. Famous North American humorist. Author. Able to sense what was in the mail.	1835–1910	33, 50
Vageler	Paul, Dr. Physical chemist in Addis Ababa. Supporter of telepathy.	Contemporary (1922)	25, 46
Vasse	Paul, M.D. G.P. in Amiens (Somme). From 1946 onwards	Contemporary	53

attempted the "forced"
growth of seedlings by
concentrated thought.

VELDENPLAN	Johann. Swedish professor of music and "simple life" reformer. Ran a "scientific bureau" in Echterdingen (Württemberg).	Contemporary	47
VIANNEY	Jean-Baptiste Marie. The "Curé d'Ars" (in Dombe; Dép.: Ain). Beatified in 1905, canonized in 1925. Feast day: August 4. Mind-reader, clairvoyant.	1786–1859	137
VIGNES	Cyprien. French thaumaturge (Theurgist) in Vialas (Lozère).	Died 1908	134
DE VILLIERS DE L'ISLE-ADAM	Philippe Auguste Mathias. Count. French writer.	1840–1889	117
VÖLGYESI	Franz (Ferenc), M.D. Well-known medical hypnotist in Budapest. Writer.	Born 1895	2, 26, 28, 116
VÖLLER	Walther, M.D., Ph.D. Medical Superintendent of the "Convalescent Home for Encephalitis Patients" in Kassel- Harleshausen. Studies in organic electricity.	1893–1954	2, 13, 36

W.	J. Young girl who was a spiritual healer in Watkins, NY. Known to Dr. Franz HARTMANN.	1888	52
WAGNER	Christian. Swabian peasant poet.	1835–1862	144
WALTHER	Gerda, Ph.D. Well-known parapsychologist and writer in Munich. *Phänomenologie der Mystik* [The Phenomenology of Mysticism] (2nd Edition: 1955).	Born 1897	104, 106
WEININGER	Canadian psychologist of German origin, special-izing in the nervous diseases of children.	Contemporary	141
WELISCH	Ludwig. Central school head teacher in Graz; even-tually school inspector there. Pendulum researcher. Friend of SURYA.	1876–1945	41, 42
WERINOS	W., Dr. Bioclimatologist in Graz.	Contemporary (1956)	73
WICKLAND	Carl A., M.D. Mental specialist in Los Angeles, CA. Adherent of the possession theory in psychoses with no organic cause.	1862–1937	136
WILLIAM OF PARIS	*Guillaume de Paris;* also *Guillaume d'Auvergne.*	1180–1249	49

	Bishop of Paris from 1228. Real-philosophical works.		
WILKINS	George Hubert, Sir. Polar aviator.	1888–1958	37
WIMMER	August, M.D. Professor of Psychiatry in the University of Copenhagen and Medical Superintendent of the Psychiatric and Neurological Hospital there.	Born 1872	74
WOJNOWSKI	Oskar, Ph.D. Medical herbalist; diagnosed by laying on of hands.	1926	17
WOLTON	Henry. Prominent person in Saratoga Springs, NY. Host of Joseph BONAPARTE.	1825	29
WÜST	Joseph., M.D., Ph.D. Physicist and parapsychologist in Munich. Specially commendable for the elucidation of telepathy, Od, dowsing, and earth radiations.	Contemporary	99, 100
X	Madame. Pseudonym of a French medium who worked with scientists and concentrated on mummifying things with the hands.	1912	48
YEATS-BROWN	Francis, Sir. English major, observed the aureole in yogis.	1886–1944	95

INDEX

N
narcotics, 147
neck, nape of, 31
neurogamy, 51, 94
news agency, telepathic, 37
Nirvana, 142

O
objects
   mentally charging, 113
   peripheral effect on dead, 118
ocular rays, 2, 54
Od, 12, 20, 23, 53, 54, 95, 96, 79, 105,
   110
   carriers, 22, 24
   engrams, in, 92
   Od is not, 93
   rediscovery of, 21
   vampires, 47
odic
   exhalations, 115
   jammers, 43
   phenomena, 46
odically deficient, 18
odor of sanctity, 5
organ, parietal, 32
organic neurosis, 61
organoelectrometer, 2

P
Pak Subuh, 117
passes
   distant, 19
   positive, 22
pearls, anemic, 24
pendant, 22
pendulum, 41, 42, 114
   experiments, 40
penetration, unusual sensory, 74
people, psychoactive, 1
persona, 76
Pfeiffer's crystallization diagnosis, 88
Phantom limb pains, 102
Philippe phenomenon, 128
physical

ailments, 62
   presence, influenced by, 1
pictures, positive mental, 56
Pitta currents, 112
plants, 83
poison, emotional, 85
polypsychismus, 73
possession, 136
postures, sprawling, 18
Pranayama, 93, 95
prayer, 136, 146
   to evoke Brahma, 55
Psi-gamma abilities, 146
Psi-pi-phenomenon, ix
psychic
   dynamides, 112
   impulse, 110
   reflex waves, 75
psychic energy, negative
   from inanimate objects and dis-
      turbed areas, 118–125
psychogenic
   autointoxication, 85
   autotoxins, 74
psychometry, 113

R
radiation, 6, 95
   indicator, 42
radioactivity, 89
Ram Das, ix
Rauwolfia serpentina, 147
regenerative impulse, 58
relics, 23
remedies, homeopathic, 87
resonance, 46
rheumatism, 59
rhinitis vasomotoria, 59
ring, magic, 42
Rosicrucians, 102

S
sahala, 53
saliva, 87

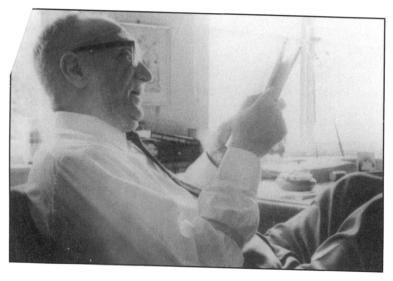

Willy Schrödter (1897–1971) was a businessman and also served as a councilor in the German government. He spent his mature years studying and researching serious esoteric subjects. His notes have proven to be invaluable references.